BREAK UP ASCENSION

How to Transform Your Breakup Into Your Spiritual Awakening with the Power of Acceptance and Forgiveness

by Saskia Kalwinek

© 2025 by Saskia Kalwinek

All rights reserved.

No portion of this book may be reproduced in any form without written permission from the author, except as permitted by Australian copyright law. For permissions contact: info@loveempowermentclinic.com.au

This publication is designed to provide accurate and authoritative information in regard to the subject matter covered. It is sold with the understanding that the author is not engaged in rendering legal, investment, accounting, or other professional services. While the author has used their best efforts in preparing this book, she makes no representations or warranties with respect to the accuracy or completeness of the contents of this book and specifically disclaim any implied warranties of merchantability or fitness for a particular purpose. No warranty may be created or extended by sales representatives or written sales materials. The advice and strategies contained herein may not be suitable for your situation. You should consult with a professional when appropriate. The author will not be liable for any loss of profit or any commercial damages, including but not limited to special, incidental, personal, or other damages.

Book Cover and eBook Formatting by Saskia Kalwinek
Edited by
1st Edition 2024

eBook ISBN: 978-1-7635798-4-2
Hard Cover ISBN: 978-1-7635798-5-9
Paperback ISBN: 978-1-7635798-6-6
Audiobook ISBN: 978-1-7635798-7-3

Visit the author's website at www.loveempowermentclinic.com.au

Contents

ACKNOWLEDGEMENTS 5

FOREWORD 7

Chapter One: Cut the Cords Properly 11

Chapter Two: Be Still and Regulate 25

Chapter Three: Establish a Healthy Routine 31

Chapter Four: Dealing with Ruminations 39

Chapter Five: Don't Overstimulate
with Fixes – keep your mind on the game 51

Chapter Six: Don't Under Stimulate
and Process Your Emotions 73

Chapter Seven: Craft Pain into Creativity 79

Chapter Eight: Use Fluctuations in Attachment Style
to Your Advantage 93

Chapter Nine: Address Your Generational Trauma 111

Chapter Ten: Signs that You Are Healing 121

Chapter Eleven: Signs that You Are Ready
to Get Back Out There 133

AFTERWORD 145

References 147

ACKNOWLEDGEMENTS

I would like to thank my family and friends for staying by my side and helping me through life, listening to my problems, and witnessing my sadness, pain, but also happiness, excitement, and all other emotions. During this time, I learned not to have expectations, and that gives me so much more gratitude and brings more love and connection into my life. With this book, I would like to express and explore what true love and connection mean so that after those breakups, we all can find something genuine and fulfilling.

I would also like to thank all of my ex-partners and even other short-term romantic connections for teaching me how to be humble, speak my truth, and eventually understand what love means.

FOREWORD

It's never easy to say goodbye to someone with whom you had hoped you'd be in a long-lasting relationship, especially when feeling overwhelmed with love for that person. Those feelings of loss can sometimes rip our psyche apart and even manifest physically. After all, emotional pain is, in fact, a form of physical pain. And anyone who has experienced pain wastes no time looking for relief. Some end up hyper-focused on the person, mistaking them as the only cure for their heartache, rather than focusing on the healing process. Whereas others, in haste, focus on escaping their pain, mistaking that as a shortcut for their healing.

Now, of course, there are those who are less affected and are less prone to seeking extremes, having little difficulty falling back into their old routines. These individuals may have less of a need for this book. However, there are others who aren't entirely honest with themselves and may try to overcompensate and project an image that they are doing better with their situation than they truly are.

When this is the case, some may tend to over-socialize or avoid socializing altogether when experiencing such pain. While over-socializing might cover up your emotions and compartmentalise the pain, it runs the risk of escaping into the emotions of others and further destabilising our own psyche, rather than taking the proper time to heal and reflect.

Another example would be increased alcohol consumption, which is an escapism rather than a path to healing and more often replaces one type of trauma to your body with another. Not only do such behaviours negatively impact you emotionally, they will damage your metabolism, your digestive system, your immune system, and create increased inflammation in the brain.

Another extreme might take the form of excessive exercise, eating disorders, excessive running, or other types of harsh cardio, all of which can negatively affect a person's health, joints, and connective tissues, among other health concerns. To everything, there must be a balance. Without balance, every activity not only offers the potential of some sort of release but also carries the risk of a variety of problems. The only healthy way to move on is to give an equal amount of attention to each part of your life and not overdo any one activity, especially when approached as an escape, which should never be mistaken for healing.

Moving on should likewise not be mistaken for healing. If you're seeing someone new and find yourself still missing your ex or carrying feelings of anger, those feelings will arise in any new relationship for as long as those feelings go unaddressed and until you finally devote the time and space to healing, to clearing your mind, addressing your pain, your false hopes, and limiting beliefs.

This book is meant to serve you as a guide for helping you move through that unpleasant experience as swiftly and safely as possible. Through a fusion of psychological and spiritual techniques, I will accompany you on this journey.

What You'll Uncover in the Pages Ahead

Through this book, we'll cover the initial phase of a breakup—such as how to communicate after the ending of the relationship, and boundaries that need to be established. Then we'll take the first steps towards the healing process—accepting the emotions and pain that comes flooding in. We'll learn how to adopt self-regulation and how to properly conduct our inner dialogue with our inner voices, where the different parts within us are making conflicting demands. We will define healthy routines and how to reconcile our ruminations through this period of distress. From there, we'll discuss additional preventative measures—such as not over or under-stimulating yourself—so that you can safely conclude your healing journey. After this, you'll arrive at the most difficult time of the break-up—the bittersweet channeling of your pain into creativity and manifesting goodness in your life.

Along the way, we'll examine how releasing transgenerational traumas can cut attachment cords with certain people in your life.

In the final chapters, I will reveal how to recognize whether your healing process is underway, and how you'll know whether you're ready to reengage in the dating world. Lastly, we will talk about how to use the lessons from this painful period in your future relationships and in life in general.

Honestly, this timeline may differ from person to person, depending on the intensity, toxicity, and duration of a relationship. For example, my most recent experience took 4 months. That process was extremely intense, in both good and toxic ways. At the beginning of that relationship, we'd both felt we'd met each other's equal in all ways. It was an intense experience for both of us, but in both of our cases, our personal work was incomplete. He often became avoidant, shying away from the intensity, whereas I became preoccupied and held expectations I wasn't communicating. In the end, he chose not to do the emotional work with me, which resulted in a much-needed reality check.

In hindsight, I am grateful for the personal transformation that followed, which wouldn't have happened if he had chosen to stay and do the work. I had already stayed in that situation for far too long. In the end, I realised the work I needed to do, which I'll go into more detail on later.

In this book, I'll present multiple healing techniques and exercises, and together we'll sculpt your pain into learning, creation, and love, breaking the cycle of generating more pain. Similar to an uncleansed wound resulting in an infection, negative energy will always take on another shape or form without proper healing.

In the back of this book, I will offer references to more reading material pertaining to some of the pioneers of the techniques I've incorporated into my approach. I'll also offer further resources for escaping abusive relationships and where to seek help and legal aid.

No matter what your situation is, you are not alone, and I'll help you analyze your patterns in the breakups and relationships you've experienced, just as I have mine. I can help you make sense of the anger and feelings of injustice. I will help you reach a sense of peace with your independence rather than feeling crippled by loss and loneliness. That liberating independence can be ever-present once you are able to let go of every perceived transgression in your relationships, which often continues long after a break-up.

So buckle up for work ahead if you're serious about getting over your ex!

Chapter One: Cut the Cords Properly

Before you can enter the healing process, you need to cut ties and limit your contact with your ex as much as possible. This is not something you can do together. It doesn't matter if you've committed to maintaining a friendship, are remaining open to getting back together in the future, or still have some joint responsibilities. For as long as you stay in regular contact, you will not heal or change for the better.

For many, this can feel painful and difficult to initiate. You may justify not taking such action, rationalizing being civil and thinking practically about these things is the proper approach. However, you need to remember this isn't about practicality. It is a matter of the heart. If you don't get this part right, you run the risk of encountering problems later that will prevent you from healing and growth.

Think of this as "breakup administration". It is about preparing for your journey towards a new you, which means forming new habits, establishing boundaries, and practicing healthy values, all towards prioritising everything else in your life. And you can't focus on you when you are focused on that other person.

What Qualifies Me To Write This Book?

I am an accredited sex therapist, counselor, a couples' therapist, an Internal Family System (IFS) therapist, and I also specialize in Relational

Life Therapy (RLT). Both IFS and RLT share similar features, which I will go into greater depth on in the coming pages. For example, there is the Functional Adult state and the Adaptive Child state.

In a Functional Adult state, we are capable of making good decisions, thinking logically and objectively, and having the best communication. The Adaptive Child state uses a different Part of the brain, the Functional Adult state, which evolved before we became human during evolution. This Part of the brain is commonly referred to as the "reptilian brain"; it's a very instinctual and preservation mechanism-oriented Part of us. When reacting from the Adaptive Child mindset, we're likely to fight, flight, or freeze instead of acting with courage, or practicing strong communication, and using our problem-solving skills. In the Adult state, however, we use a logical "human brain", called the Relational Brain.

Then there are those Internal Parts that exist within each of us, such as inner critics, perfectionists, withdrawers, and others that make us act or think in certain ways. These conceal difficult emotions such as shame, hurt, or fear, and those are referred to as Exile Parts. Those Parts are similar in nature to the Adaptive Child state. However, they can be eased and unburdened through connection with Self Energy, which is who we are at the core. In our Self Energy mode, we are courageous, calm, creative, and curious, so for me this state corresponds with the Adult brain.

In this book, I'll frequently explore our adult state, or the Kid/Child state, and dive deeper into the various other *parts of us*. I'll introduce the concept that we should uncover what those parts of us need and try to fulfill them in a healthy and mature way. For example, if your angry Part wants respect from others, it may communicate this by lashing out. However, a healthier way of addressing those needs would be to openly demand respect from others. Or if your people-pleaser Part wants you to keep the peace between you and a loved one, you can establish healthy boundaries that will help you voice your needs while keeping the peace in alignment with your values.

I also use techniques such as Cognitive Behavioural Therapy, Art Therapy, and Schema Therapy. These modalities help me understand my clients and challenge them to change their mindsets while improving their lives. With these approaches, and others, I've helped my clients better express themselves, understand what they need and want, how to self-analyse their thoughts and behaviours, of making sense of them, while channeling healthier habits, such as through artistic expression.

Apart from my vast psychological and coaching knowledge, I also have a lot of real-world personal experience as well. I have been there, having learned many lessons firsthand through my own relationships. I am intimately familiar with several types of attachment styles, from being avoidant, fearful, secure, and preoccupied. Each depended on the type of partner I was with at the time.

Then I went through a break-up like no other. My emotional pain manifested physically in the final weeks of that relationship. It felt like someone else was inside of my head. I realised again that my insecurities, issues with boundaries, low self-esteem, jealousy, and other unhelpful patterns were no longer needed. I'd worked on all those issues previously, and their residual energies reemerged in that relationship. There were so many emotions I needed to release at the same time. That's when I decided I had to do all the work at once or my symptoms would continue to magnify.

So I dove into excessive meditation, which led me to discovering Kundalini Energy. That's when I decided to conduct an experiment. I wanted to test how quickly I could recover from that breakup. This is not typically recommended for those who don't have enough of a social support, a good routine, healthy habits, or a secure life situation in place. However, I rationalised that my life was set up in a way that made it easy for me to isolate myself for a couple of weeks and just focus on the work.

At first, I dove too deeply into it before learning to pace myself and eventually master it. During Kundalini Awakening, people emotionally and physically purge, kind of like having a mental breakdown but with breaks for extreme bliss and increased pleasure. You get very emotional, but you come back from it to experience life in a new and improved way. However, when you rush it, and don't trust the process, it's common to get stuck in some of the emotions you are trying to process, which results in what is called the "Dark Knight of Kundalini Awakening".

Going slow and steady did not interest me. So I set out on my experiment, deciding I wanted to feel the full gravity of my emotions and do it the hardcore way. I knew the steps. I started in on my intense meditations. My awakening arrived swiftly, but was extremely difficult and painful. My body opened up with the Kundalini Energy, which meant muscle pains and intense waves of emotions.

As I started to experience these difficulties, I decided that perhaps it was supposed to happen at that intense pace, as I'm an intense individual and was determined to continue. So, I embraced it and felt pride for how much I could endure. At first, my body started purging so strongly that I had difficulties with keeping food and water in. This lasted for days. Soon I had difficulty sleeping. My heart was racing and my depression and anxiety increased. This lasted for weeks.

Finally, I found my Reiki Practitioner and mentor, Alex Robibaro, who helped me normalise and get rid of excess energy from my body. By no means was I done. I knew all the tricks in the book on how to do it, so I locked myself up for over a week and conducted an express recovery. I had to let everything in, acknowledge my part in it, forgive him and myself. Admittedly, the pain was excruciating for the first few days, but I felt better pretty quickly. I still experienced body aches because of the awakening, but got used to stronger energies moving through my body. I also moved them by myself and released them with understanding. I graduated through the extreme sense of loss and anger, and was left with some sadness, but greater hope for a future reconnection. Eventually, the fear of loneliness decreased, and I was able to enjoy what I had created on this painful journey.

In the midst of that, I managed to discover my parental wounds, heal them, and achieve a better connection with people in my life. I also found a better and more fulfilling way of living and running my company. This type of extreme breakup work requires a lot of emotional courage and time.

Through this fusion of psychological and spiritual modalities, I will walk with you. I'll share my own stories, and those of friends and family, what we've learned from them, and how you can apply those lessons to yourself, and demonstrate how dramatically different each unique situation can be.

There are two kinds of boundaries. External boundaries are those we create with other people. And internal boundaries are those we create within ourselves.

With external boundaries, rather than creating a safe space for ourselves, we make requests of how others are to be when they are around us. No matter how kindly we communicate them, such requests must be made with an acceptance that people will not always adhere to them. And when our expectations are not met, we need to be flexible, and either adapt or politely remove ourselves from the company of that person as a last resort.

Now, think of internal boundaries as a set of rules that are driven by your values in life. This is how you might define what "being a good person" looks like to you. What does it mean to be a good daughter or a son? What does it mean to be a good mother or a father? What does it mean to be a good coworker, employee, or boss?

The answers to these questions aren't always straightforward. Primarily, you want to be true and compassionate not only to yourself but also to others. You need to find balance and shift your perspective of the world. Perceive yourself as equal to everyone else, and not above or below others. When you truly hold yourself in the same regard as you hold others, your self-esteem will improve. Striking a healthy balance to your self-esteem is crucial for developing boundaries and re-establishing your values.

Finding clarity in what you value in your life will offer focus on what behaviors adhere to your set of internal rules, resulting in establishing healing habits. For example, showing love to yourself and to others through valuing a healthy lifestyle, which translates to regular exercise, and a balanced nutrition-focused diet.

EXERCISE 1
Values → Boundaries → Habits

A. Write down what you presently value in life and what you are aspiring towards.
B. Write down what external and internal boundaries you want to form with others that offer protection and that follow those values.
C. Write down those habits you want to form, which will help you live in line with those values.

EXERCISE 2
Boundary Wall

Next, we are going to imagine putting up a boundary wall around you. This following technique will help you actively protect yourself in a diplomatic way in vulnerable situations, and is especially useful when applied in all instances of "breakup administration". It can also help you stop internalizing (taking things personally), externalizing (blaming others, environment, or external circumstances), imposing your view on others, and others from imposing their views on you.

First, imagine a wall in front of you. I prefer a glass wall, but it can be made of anything you want: cotton candy, flowers, brick, etc. Next, imagine this wall has a window through which you can clearly see your former partner. Now, imagine that person says something that imposes their will upon you, or something you disagree with, or something that would normally be upsetting or even hurtful. But, instead of those statements and words penetrating you, they instead hit the wall. Whether they stick to this wall or bounce off of it is up to you. But the words are now in front of you and you can observe them at a comfortable distance and form your own objective opinion about what they are communicating to you.

Instead of internalising or externalising, try to objectify these things and actively listen to what they are truly communicating before you respond. Observing their opinions in this manner will protect you from feeling pressured into adopting their opinions as your own. Then you can offer your perspective and feel safer when expressing an opinion that differs from theirs.

But this wall is intended to protect them as well. It will remind you, for the same reason, not to impose your feelings upon that other person, and not to say anything rude or cruel that is counter-productive to your healing. So, anytime you start to feel stressed, or are worried a difficult topic might arise, practice putting up your boundary wall. This will aid you in becoming more flexible, adaptable, and a more skilled conversationalist. Remember, a decent debater may state their perspective, whereas a great one can examine multiple perspectives and present their viewpoint from multiple angles.

Never feel obligated to agree with what other people say. When hearing other people's opinions, accept them as something that belongs to them and not to you. Choosing to listen and not respond is often preferable to agreeing when you don't. Also, you don't always have to disagree, or stir the pot for argument's sake. There is greater empowerment in letting go.

Breaking Up With An Abusive Partner

This type of breakup requires keeping your wits about you. Your safety comes first, and the safety of your kids. Therefore, it's important to exercise as much precaution as necessary depending on how abusive or violent you believe your partner may potentially be. Anything that has happened before in an abusive relationship has a statistical probability of happening again, so never take a period of peaceful relations for granted, nor trust their word that there won't be any more difficult situations ahead.

On the other extreme, sometimes abuse can take the form of an extremely controlling partner who is taking measures to keep you from leaving, such as guarding or monitoring your phone, or invading and taking away your privacy. Breakups induce strong feelings for both parties, and there is no telling what the other person is going to do or how they may try to prevent you from leaving if they suspect it.

Sometimes that requires getting another phone, there are organisations who can provide you with one in such situations, which I reference in the back of this book, along with other resources you can turn to in such situations. (Australian Government 2024 & 2025; Uniting Communities 2024; Wesley Mission 2025; Wesnet 2025) Make sure you don't leave any important documents or essentials behind before conducting the breakup. Sometimes it means a restraining order, sometimes moving to a new location, and sometimes you won't need these things. Some other precautions could include contacting a lawyer, domestic violence center, and police before leaving so that you have a legal trial in case anything goes wrong.

Plan carefully and don't make any rash decisions. Leaving straight away isn't always the safest option. If you can gather the financial resources, you'll need to make a safe exit, do so, and make sure you have a strong social support in place as well. It's important to have a plan in place to prevent any possible violent situations, such as informing friends and family, and having people you trust be present with you when you leave.

It's also okay if you do not want to do it face-to-face. This process can ensure that cutting ties is as swift as possible and that you will not need to deal with these things later. In any case, planning is essential.

Breaking Up With a Narcissistic Partner

By narcissistic I don't necessarily mean someone with a Narcissistic Disorder, which accounts for only 1% of the population. Rather, I am referring to those grandiose individuals who resort to playing mind games, gaslighting, badmouthing, who generally aim to draw you into their toxicity.

There is honestly no nice way to split with a narcissistic person. With these individuals, it is always important to be prepared for some sort of backlash. Narcissistic partners often try to provoke reactions. They interpret reactions as emotions, and evoking emotions means control. The truth is, the emotions and patterns of others do affect us, and we need to take that into account.

No matter how tempting it may be in those situations to tell them exactly what you think of them, compose yourself. Recognize that if you want a swift break, you'll need to minimize any unpleasantries. You are in control of you, so don't give them satisfaction. Maintain your values and your boundaries.

Being the bigger person isn't always easy. But in doing so, you'll be creating peace of mind for yourself. So try not to engage. Go into practical mode, whether you are about to break up with them, or immediately after they break up with you. Think about what needs to be done, picked up, wrapped up, or settled. Emotional control is crucial if you want to stop the cycle of pain. Try to disengage. Give them the space to feel whatever they need to feel while protecting yourself with boundaries. Aim for as little contact as possible.

I once broke up with a partner with narcissistic traits who I also happened to work with. After the breakup, he started gossiping and badmouthing me to our coworkers and our boss. The more I focused my positive attention on my work and my working relationships without being emotionally drawn into his tactics, the more he would try to provoke me verbally in front of others. Eventually, his behavior and lack of emotional self-control spoke for itself, and the people we worked with saw the situation for what it was. Counter a Narcissist with your emotional regulation and they will dig their own grave or lose interest.

Breaking Up With a Partner Who Lacks Boundaries

It's human to feel confused in situations where emotions are heightened. Confused people confuse other people. Even I, the author of this book, consider myself to be a fairly level-headed person. I typically know exactly what I want and how I want it.

Nevertheless, in one relationship with a person whom I shared a deep connection with, there was a great deal of confusion over what he wanted. During those four months, I lost my objectivity, and gradually my commonsense, as I increasingly felt gaslighted and questioned my own sanity. When I raised valid questions, he'd accuse me of "overthinking" things. He'd also frequently redirect the conversation towards himself and express "being afraid to get hurt".

Often, these avoidance techniques would shut down any deeper conversations or reaching any real answers. Eventually, I decided these tactics weren't working for me. So I started over-giving in the relationship while evaluating his responses to my increased investment in the relationship. This eventually led to me deeming it necessary to vocally communicate that I needed a commitment.

He responded by telling me that this was too confusing and overwhelming for him. That's when I realised he couldn't give me the relationship that I wanted, so I left. His avoidance felt like a rejection, and I needed space to deal with those feelings. So I organized and gathered my belongings. Reflecting on our avoidant vs. pursuer dynamic, I wrote a goodbye message to him, communicating that I'd accepted his decision.

I'd reached a place of clarity, and the confusion was dispelled. When ending a relationship with a partner who has difficulties with people-pleasing holds little regard for your boundaries, it requires calm objectivity. And, once I regained that clarity and was able to detach myself, he sent another confusing message, expressing how he misses me, that he is all broken up over it, and wants to talk to me face to face. At first, it was difficult for me to imagine him suffering. Yet, I soon found myself entertaining what a future together would look like, and my objectivity was, yet again, soon lost. I found myself changing my mind every five minutes. Yet, I knew I couldn't repeat our previous pattern.

Eventually, I decided the right thing to do in that situation was to tell him if he wanted to meet, I would only see him to talk about what happened, and define the conditions I would require to consider getting back together. That was when he repeated his behavior of avoidance and didn't respond. Then he'd reach out again in a similar fashion, and we went around and around in circles for two weeks.

Even though I maintained my position and set boundaries, I found myself emotionally handicapped and unable to do anything other than watch TV and eat my feelings. Finally, he ended up dropping off my things, and we said our final goodbyes. There were no hard feelings. I think fondly of him and consider him a good soul. Yet, the amount of turmoil he created was significant. All because he refused to connect to his feelings, and in his confusion, I lost track of my feelings and boundaries in the name of infatuation. When I was in a state of wanting that relationship with him, I prioritised those wants over my needs. What I needed was to regain sanity and look after myself.

It is important to make decisions based on what you need rather than what you want. If you find yourself in a similar situation, I recommend reaching a state of calm through physical exercise and through breathwork. Find your Functional Adult in the middle of it all and channel that objective Part of your mind. Look at the other parts as just voices calling for help. You can look after and address those voices yourself. You already have everything you need.

You don't need to look to your ex to come and save you. What is it that you believe they have that you need? Once you discover what that is, you'll realize it is something that you can give to yourself. Once you do that, the attachment will fade. This was my favorite mantra when I started to ruminate again; "Everything I need, I have here with me."

Breaking Up With a Secure Partner

This is the best type of breakup one can hope for. A relationship that was mostly secure and ends due to a difference in values or diverting life paths typically results in a clean break. When it makes sense to a couple why they should no longer be together, there's typically strong communication, open feelings, and respected boundaries. They are nicer to each other, and usually there is little to no resentment or anger. That's not to say because there is no damage, there isn't a sense of loss. It's just remarkably different from the pain, turmoil, and damage that results from a toxic relationship.

Final Message/Letter/Chat

Less communication is recommended the more toxic and abusive a relationship is. An abusive or narcissistic partner is less likely to consider what you have to say. In these situations, it is human to want closure, validation, or to be understood and feel justified for leaving. However, it's important to remember that frequently partners mirror one another. We teach each other about our flaws and often reflect them back throughout our personal development. Breakups often result in breakthroughs, revealing things about ourselves that were previously hidden. I've learned a lot about myself through every relationship I've had and grown from it.

If you do want to be that final mirror, let it reflect love. Gather as much kindness as you can. It's impossible, as a human being, to have wholly pure intentions. But we can each of us do our best. Admittedly, I often mirror in part to feel better about myself. Yes, I am genuinely concerned for those I've been in relationships with, and to a degree concerned for their prospective future partners. I believe when we are able to communicate in difficult situations such as these, it is better to do so with love and kindness as often as we can.

Silence often isn't kind. It can prolong the problem and the pain. Some might not be ready for your truth, and that's okay. Others will take what you share and forge that into growth and self-development. Nevertheless, we also need to acknowledge when we've gone too far and become unproductive when it comes to our final remarks in a relationship. Always weigh the pros and cons. Look after yourself, and weigh the consequences and potential backlash of voicing that final truth.

Maintaining Radio Silence

When everything that needs to be said is said, and all your affairs are in order, it's important not to reengage when there's no hope for a serious reconciliation. Keeping in touch and looking at each other's stories and social media is not going to help you either. If you still harbor any feelings, you'll want to rethink this strategy. Even if you eventually reengage in a friendly way at some point, it won't be completely honest if you don't give yourself the time and space to grieve and process your emotions. Rarely are people so self-aware, developed, or at peace with a breakup straight after it happens. For those who have Messiah-like forgiveness and acceptance abilities, by all means, continue the contact. For the rest of us, it's important to be honest with ourselves.

When this support system is ripped away from you, your brain is in turmoil because all the dopamine related to your relationship is gone and you go into withdrawal. Infatuation is like a drug, from which we are rewarded with validation, security, sex, and connection. And there is no potent enough substitute for it. That's why people often spiral into bad habits straight after. You wouldn't invite a one-day sober alcoholic into a bar. You need sufficient time for radio silence from this person in order to be able to pick yourself up and tend to your needs.

Chapter Two:
Be Still and Regulate

This next chapter is all about learning how to center ourselves amidst the turmoil we may be experiencing. It's important to acknowledge that we're still in the beginning phase. During this phase, it's easy to fall back into escapism, overstimulation, and a lack of self-regulation. It is as important as ever during this period to stay true to our values and avoid the toxic coping strategies we may have turned to in the past. And if we slip up now and again, that's okay. We all make mistakes and we all want to escape our suffering.

Remember when I shared my negative experience taking kundalini meditation to an extreme? Instead of exercising moderation and constantly re-centering myself while practicing my measured breathing, I found myself enjoying drifting off into it so much; it turned into an escape and became hard for me to stop. So, if you too find that you've been escaping, and find yourself challenged by stillness and self-regulation, here are some exercises that will help you reach the calmness that's been evading you.

EXERCISE 3
Centering Touch

Throughout the day, any time you feel some difficult sensations or troubling thoughts arising, try to comfort yourself and address your primary fears, such as a common fear of loneliness, fear of dying (alone), or fear of rejection. There are a myriad of emotions we may be struggling with in these situations, but most of them lead to some variety of fear or shame.

So, when you find yourself struggling with these self-afflicting emotions, practice reassuring yourself. Gently touch your leg, arm, or belly. Pet yourself a bit as you center your thoughts and refocus on your body. Through this practice, you'll learn to straddle the spiritual side and the real world. You'll be bringing something physical and real together with something that is wholly yours, manifesting your internal world.

EXERCISE 4
Values Check

The following exercise is intended to help you hone your understanding of what being a good, responsible person, partner, daughter, son, friend—means to you. Approaching being honest, kind, and having a balanced life through a healthy and mindful calmness is not only healing, but gives us purpose. So, to prepare, gather something to write with, and a notebook or journal to write in.

A. Start by making a list of your values. These are things you aspire to embody in your ideal self. They are the boundaries which inform your habits, thoughts, and behaviors on the path to becoming a better human being. So, ask yourself: "When am I at my best mental capacity, how would I describe my ideal of a good person?"

B. Next, find time each day to think about and write down anything that didn't feel aligned with your values since your last entry. Next, beside each example, write down what you think you can do better to be more aligned with the person you are striving to be. Try to make a practice of notating your progress. Anytime you identify moments where you were aligned with your values and best practices in your life, take pride in those accomplishments.

Behavioral Contagion

It is quite common to pick up the behaviors, views, emotions, and communication styles of those we are in relationships with. Although sometimes this enmeshment can be healthy, in other situations it can have a negative impact on us as well. In fact, how the behavior and emotions of those we are close to impact us can be greater than we care to admit or even realize. The more we open ourselves up to that person, and the greater the need to connect with them, the more vulnerable we are to these phenomena.

At the end of a relationship, it is more important than ever to be aware of this, as you may unknowingly possess a great deal of your "ex's energy" inside of you. This is not only a spiritual component, but a psychological one as well. This can lead to inner conflict similar to what we've experienced in that last relationship, despite not being with them anymore, and can carry negative consequences into our future relationships as well.

Imagine you dated someone who was a people pleaser, yet had difficulty acknowledging their emotions, and often felt overwhelmed by them. This created difficult-to-pinpoint issues throughout the relationship. Now imagine, unknowingly, you started doing the same thing around him. Eventually, you stopped trying to address your issues and compartmentalised your emotions because they weren't being received or understood. At first, that partner seemed like a person with no problems, and you admired that and naturally tried to mirror it. However, as problems between you arose, you eventually stopped expressing yourself from, somehow, in an effort to try to please them.

After the relationship ended, in a moment of honesty and self-reflection, you recognised those uncomfortable traits within you. This then led to feelings of shame for losing a sense of your identity and independence. Not believing yourself to ever be insecure in a relationship, you struggled to identify when this crept up on you and how it has affected other parts of your life. You then realise how that insecurity impacted your relationships with your friends and family as well.

X-ENERGY

It's easy to experience a brief loss of trust in yourself while entertaining a toxic relationship. This is what I mean by carrying your *ex's energy* with you. So, before you can heal, you need to assess what is yours and what is theirs. Try to identify any negatives you've picked up from them. It can be a bad habit, like excessive drinking or smoking or an unhealthy diet. It could be through antisocial behaviors or trust issues and a negative outlook.

Examine every aspect of who you are being now versus who you were before you met that person. What do you want to keep and what do you need to leave behind? Have you adopted any affectations, perceptions, outlooks, or beliefs that aren't functional or that you wouldn't be proud of? These need to be addressed in order to move on. Otherwise, you'll likely start to assign blame for being that way, without rebuilding your confidence and strengthening and reinforcing your emotional systems.

Going deeper, the fact that you adopted and carried that *ex's energy* with you, it is important to recognise they were just a catalyst for some unaddressed energy and emotions that were dormant inside of you. This is what caused you to adopt their behaviour instead of preserving strong boundaries. Your *ex's energy* was a placeholder for the self-esteem you were seeking at the time.

EXERCISE 5
Energetic Reboot

Remain focussed on your breathing. Softly breathing in and gently breathing out. Now imagine a pyramid of calming white light in the sky directly above you. It is descending and slowly encompasses your entire body. You feel safe, as if this white light is protecting you from everything in the universe. The energy it gives you is positive and warm, rendering sensations of security and belonging.

Concentrate on those feelings of safety and belonging. Meditate on what that feels like, and where you feel it in your body? Does it come in waves? How would you describe those sensations? What images come to mind in association with these feelings? Is it a fantasy, or perhaps a memory? As soon as you discover what your representation of safety is, *anchor it* within you. Do whatever you need to ensure you remember it and can return to it later.

Now, as you continue to visualize this pyramid of safety and illumination, pay attention to your emotions. See what feelings are joining you? Recognize them as your own, or as those emotions that belong to others. If you are not sure, ask yourself who they belong to, and listen to the answers that come. Then, as soon as they are identified, release those emotional burdens that don't belong to you and let them be carried up and away from you into the light. These are their belongings, not yours, and it is time to pack them up and give them back. When you let go of them, and release them, do so not with anger or sadness, but with acceptance, understanding, and compassion.

At the beginning of the healing process, this can be especially difficult to do. If you find this difficult, don't let shame or other insecurities in. Be kind to yourself and do what you can. Calm acceptance is just one part of the healing process. Although it sounds easy, even this can take practice. But it starts by trusting yourself to feel safe with yourself. Regularly practicing this exercise will accustom you to this mental shift, and it will become easier for you to change those behaviors.

When you are able to release your *ex's energy*, focus on what's left. What percentage of those emotions and behaviors belong to you? Remaining calm and centered, spend time with those emotions and listen. Those parts of you will voice their needs. Hear them and start feeling better. Usually, they'll tell you that they need you to go back to living in line with your values and becoming that better person you strive to be.

Find a time of day that works best for you. Personally, I recommend making this a practice at the end of each day. By not internalizing the feelings and behaviors of others, you can allow yourself to process the emotional load from any given busy day.

Making a Practice of Finding Balance

Being still and centered is the key to finding balance. The beginning is always the most difficult and painful part of the journey. Every step you take should be taken with care. Just one misstep or stumble can create more pain from which you'll then need to recover and heal. If your inner voices try to steer you in the wrong direction, express curiosity about what they are saying and why. Try to determine what they need from you in order to be less active and calm.

Too often, those voices arise from a need to escape the pain. But what's important is to question which pains those voices are stemming from. Is it the pain of loss, rejection, self-esteem, loneliness? And, are what those voices are asking for just another means of escape, which will lead to more pain and delaying your healing journey with one detour after another?

We've all at one time or another doubted whether we are good enough, and resorted to extremes to prove that voice otherwise by doing something out of the ordinary. But without healing first, this typically leads to more problems. The most important part of the healing process is doing the work whereby you can authentically reassure yourself that you are good enough and you do matter, and you don't need external validation to believe in that undeniable truth. This can be especially true when you're not necessarily doing anything that would count as extraordinary. What is important is having confidence in yourself.

Too often, we withdraw from fun activities as a coping mechanism. What's important here is recognizing what dysfunctional mode you are turning on when you experience or return to the pain. Practicing these exercises and doing the work will help you assess where that pain is coming from, what to focus on within you, and speeding up your healing journey via a calm and centered, balanced life.

Chapter Three: Establish a Healthy Routine

We need to establish different types of routines at different points in our life. There is no one size fits all. Each routine is tailored to the life we live at the time. So, at this crossroads, we are going to address two common routines a person can fall into. The Rejuvenation Routine, and The Pain Masking Pain Routine. Both can eventually deliver you to a desired effect, but are quite different in the way they react with your stress hormones. Overdoing The Pain Masking Pain Routine might require you to likewise implement The Rejuvenation Routine. But first, let's take a moment to dive into these two routines in greater depth.

Rejuvenation Routine

This routine can feel more intense and difficult to endure in the beginning, but will bring you to homeostasis quicker, decreasing your cortisol levels, thereby lowering your stress and reaching a greater state of peace and balance. I highly recommend this approach for those who are experiencing severe anxiety and feelings of helplessness. It is not so dissimilar to taking a retreat or isolating in your personal sanitarium, where you develop a program for healthy healing.

During this time, you'll prepare healthy and light cooked food. A Keto-Flex diet is proven to improve mental clarity while reducing inflammation in the brain. Therefore, I personally recommend a protein-based diet with minimal carb intake, complemented with fruit and vegetables. Additionally, organic and non-processed foods are better for eliminating your toxin-intake, which likewise reduces inflammation. Some might justify not following such restrictions because it comes with a higher price point. However, this should be weighed against the cost of your mental and physical health.

Also, avoid vegetable and seed oils. These aren't sources of healthy fats and can cause damage to our digestive systems. Where you can, substitute those with healthier options that serve as brain food, such as coconut oil or MCT oil (a type of refined coconut oil), avocado oil, ghee, butter, or tallow. If you are having stomach issues, I would recommend more collagen and bone broth, probiotics such as yogurt, kimchi, sauerkraut, apple cider vinegar, and kombucha. Fiber can sometimes hurt your digestive lining, and collagen helps heal that lining. So, if you are experiencing issues, perhaps take a break from vegetables and fruit for a bit. Linseeds—also known as flaxseed—when boiled in water create a thick healing drink as well.

There are also many seemingly healthy foods that contain unhealthy proteins, such as lectins. These can negatively impact your health when you're under stress. What is extremely important is to listen to your body—and consulting with your doctor or nutritionist—and deciding what is best for you. For many, prolonged or intermittent fasting can yield many benefits. However, everyone's metabolism is different, and it is important to find the right program for you. Sometimes extended fasting can trigger a cortisol response, increasing your stress response. This is why every routine needs to be tailored to your individual needs. So approach the suggestions in this book as inspiration for where you can take your rejuvenation routine.

I like to start my day with a glass of water with 1 spoon of apple cider vinegar and a pinch of Celtic salt. It helps to weak up the digestive system, so you process the food better. Also, make sure that you have plenty of water throughout the day. I like to add a pinch of Celtic salt to a glass of water to add some minerals that water is flushing out. Water and mineral retention can be affected by anxiety and elevated levels of cortisol. I also take plenty of supplements. I'm not qualified in that area, but researching helpful supplements is a hobby of mine. Here is a list of things that I take daily:

- Vitamin A, B12 (every second day), C, D3 with K2, E
- Fish Oil (Omega-3)
- NAC
- NMN (longevity supplement, that reverses aging)
- Sodium Butyrate (good for the digestive system)
- Creatine (helps to build muscle, building muscle is a good predictor of longevity. Don't worry ladies, it's actually very hard to get bulky.)
- Resveratrol
- Zinc
- Potassium
- Magnesium Glycinate

I suggest being careful with brands. If you buy the cheapest stuff, you will not get good results. I highly recommend Bioceuticals, Thorne, and LifeSeasons. I usually take zinc, potassium, and magnesium in the evening before I go to bed on an empty stomach. The rest I take with meals. That maximizes the intake, especially when done so with healthy fats.

I am a personal believer that combining supplements with living a more ayurvedic lifestyle is the path to achieving a greater balance between mind, body, and spirit. An unfortunate side effect of the times we live in is to be mindful of all the environment hazards to our health that are everywhere around us, even in the very food we eat. The methods used to grow and distribute crops through industrialized agriculture produce food that simply isn't as healthy as it once was. So, even when being a conscientious shopper, it's important to ensure you are supplementing your diet and getting everything your body needs for optimal mental and physical health. Nevertheless, it is up to you to decide how much you are willing to take on and how lifestyle-adaptable you feel.

When I customized my own rejuvenation routine, I performed light forms of exercise, which included daily pilates and yoga. I avoided alcohol and limited my social activities to safe and comfortable settings. I went to bed every night at the same time, developing a healthy sleep routine, limited to 7-8 hours every night. I consistently remained attentive to my emotions. I journaled from a positive mindset. I practiced affirmations. I practiced grounding exercises, which kept any anxiousness at bay. I had fortnightly therapy sessions. And I incorporated art into my routine.

At one point in my life, I often painted and drew for myself. But eventually I started doing it more for other people. As a result, it become less pleasurable, which led to abandoning it altogether. But I was eventually able to reclaim it for myself. Expressing yourself through art can have an incredibly healing effect, especially when doing it for yourself, without fear of it being judged or a need for validation or acceptance.

There is an old Polish proverb that says "to treat something like an egg". If you've survived a traumatic experience, and your routine and path to healing feels fragile, or if you are feeling fragile, be gentle and nurturing with yourself. Treat yourself with care.

The Pain Masking Pain Routine

When the pain is too great, and finding balance feels unattainable, anxiety, depression, and a cycle of masking pain through habitually unsustainable escapism runs the risk of becoming the routine. Falling into a pattern of over doing it will simply lead you back to where you began, and a need to establish The Rejuvenation Routine. However, if you must approach your healing through doing more, choose something healthy to fully immerse yourself in.

Keep in mind that if you overdo this routine, the only way will be to go back to the Rejuvenation Routine. If you want to "do more" at least make it something healthy. Approach it as a foundation for your go-to routine in a crisis situation. Some purge their emotions through rigorous physical exercise, cold exposures, or other forms of extreme physical experience as a distraction from the emotional pain, or a means to temporarily displace that pain. These can lead to healthier habits, but the emotional pain remaining unaddressed will only be masked, yet ever present. This often falls into a category of maladaptive coping mechanisms, which run the risk of potentially good habits becoming harmful. So it is important not to over do it.

It's a natural reaction to seek an escape which offers to mask our pain traumas and release pent up energy. Yet when our emotions are rampant and we don't know where to run and hide from them, we often turn to an external fix, such as illicit substances, high-intensity exercise, or other stimulation. But because the majority of our life is mundane, if you are unable to establish a healing and healthy routine, you run the risk of always chasing the elusive extremes of pleasure.

Yet, drinking more will affect you emotionally, and traumatise you physically, negatively impacting your digestive and your immune system, which affects us emotionally. Excessive running or other types of harsh cardio can likewise impact our joints and connective tissues. Over-socializing might mask your emotions and postpone the pain, and can even offer an opportunity to escape into other people's emotions when we refuse to take the time needed to reflect on our own. Any activity that offers some sort of release can bring with them their own problems. The only healthy way to move forward is to devote an equal amount of attention to each part of your life, rather than overindulging in any single type of activity.

Even when we have a good routine, there is always the risk to over-socialize, or avoid socializing altogether, when we are in pain. The same goes with physical exercise. Habits which seem healthy and produce endorphins while strengthening the body can serve as a distraction from unresolved trauma. Rather, try to look forward to particular events, but don't lose sight of what you are doing right now. Lean into other parts of your life and try to do all the things in your schedule with love, compassion, and undivided attention, and it will help you transform the way you view your routine. Instead of mindlessly waiting for the weekend, start to enjoy the in-between of escape.

Breaking a Cycle of Repeating Patterns

It's important to approach your path to healing mindfully. A person who physically trains to the end of time won't change the fact that they are performing "Sisyphus work". Focusing your energy on other types of pain is only beneficial if you are also focused on healing. The healing process will probably take longer, but in some ways could be less intense and more gentle if approached mindfully. Admittedly, I've overdone it in the past, and there is no shame in being that "egg". We all, at times, need special care. But we must remember to be gentle with ourselves when this is the case!

As children, when we get hurt, it is our first instinct to cry. So physical pain is emotional pain. Likewise, when we experience extreme emotional pain, it can manifest physically in unexpected ways. Frequently, these are correlated with hidden insecurities and unresolved childhood experiences.

Literally, everything in life inflicts some form of trauma. Often, when aiming to relieve the suffering from that trauma, we rely on varying somatic techniques, such as physical exercise. Yet, when examining this more closely, this somatic technique inflicts trauma to the body. Strength training literally rips and tears our muscles apart. This then increases blood flow and puts the body to work at healing those damaged tissues. With yoga we stretch, pushing our limits, and release, gradually making our joints more flexible. The more you poke, shake, move, and lift, the more you can release that tension. Yet stretch your limits too fast, and not pacing yourself can do real damage.

Every trauma is a blend of emotional and physical damage inflicted through different means. Additionally, dense low vibrational emotional pain often prevents our bodies from properly healing itself, and the physical damage can spread. This is why it's important to consciously opt for external stimulation that has a benefit. This approach allows you to observe what you are doing in a more clinical way and perhaps lead you to choose a better direction.

Now, examining our behavioural patterns, without doing the emotional work, we risk repeating the same situations, meeting similar people who provoke similar emotions we've felt for others before. Not before long, the trauma is rebuilt in the body. Healing begins with being more present and compassionately strengthening our relationship with ourselves.

Let's say a person was in a relationship that ended and they weren't ready to let go. Just because that person didn't want to grow in the same direction doesn't mean that person cannot grow independently on their own. This is when it is more important than ever to shift their thinking and start healing and focusing on oneself and their immediate environment. It's easy to place a great deal of emphasis on a relationship and develop a learned dependancy. But there are so many other connections we can rely on with our family and friends and other healthy relationships.

If you are a person who already had a good routine beforehand and is not prone to seeking extremes, then you will find this part very easy and soothing. People who easily fall back on their routines have much better emotional regulation. Nevertheless, this book is more so for people who have issues in that department.

Also, it's vital to remember that a routine is not a substitute or a cover-up for emotional work that you should do every day with yourself. Keeping track of how you feel and experiencing those states with calmness is crucial for personal development, a healthy self-esteem, and moving on safely from a painful breakup. I highly recommend journalling, regular check-ins, mindful exercises, drawing your emotions, and taking regular mindful breaks in your work and other activities, even if it is just taking a quick breath in between appointments or after you finish a workout. Focus on yourself. Listen to your inner voices. Question what you need versus what you want, and tend to those needs.

Chapter Four: Dealing with Ruminations

In this chapter, we are going to focus on calming your body and bring you back to a balanced state anytime time you stray into ruminating on your pain and sense of loss. This is first approached by focusing on exactly what you are experiencing and to assign the correct labels to those feelings. And, there is no better place to begin than understanding exactly what your imbalance stems from.

For starters, let's examine the label of 'love.' Unconditional true love doesn't have any concept of proximity or time. It is given without expectations and could be viewed as pure connection. Think of the love one has towards a child. This manner of love which a person experiences transcends beyond expectations of fulfilling one's needs or wants. This type of love communicates, I love all of you—the good and the bad—when we are together and when we are apart. I'll always have love for you.

This is different from universal love. A person can have love for everyone, and all life, in the world. This boils down to an attitude and perception one carries, such as someone who perceives everyone as lovely souls learning their lessons where we are all at interplay and learning from each other. Then, we come at last, to the societal idea of love, which is often confused with infatuation or intimate attraction. Infatuation says, "I like the way you make me feel and what you give me, but if you leave, my love will be taken away." This type of love can be broken and leave broken hearts in its absence. Yet, in truth, your brain is not actually grieving the loss of love. It is grieving what you lost from the dissolution of that relationship which you grew accustomed to and were dependent on.

There is a lot to be gained from the security a relationship has to offer. It can help us heal, or forget about our painful insecurities. In fact, when we are open and in a trusting relationship, we feel secure with a person we trust with our vulnerabilities. This eases our fears and provides comfort, trusting we have a teammate to accompany us into an uncertain future. Even the most secure of partners get accustomed to these feelings. We come to rely on an intimate partner. We give ourselves and we get them in return. That bond crosses the threshold of instinct and survival. Therefore, on a primal level, your life is merged and dependent on the relationship in ways, and when it is suddenly no longer there, it instinctually generates a tremendous amount of stress.

Trying to convince yourself that the relationship didn't matter won't help. Even if you are adept at convincing yourself of this, you aren't doing the work, and aren't doing yourself any favors. You'll run the risk of repeating the same patterns, and piling on the trauma. This may give off an image of strength, but that strength is only skin deep.

When I exited a four-month relationship, I trivialized it. I told myself that four months was nothing, and shrugged it off, telling everyone I was over it, and ready to move on. But what I wasn't admitting was that, at that time, I'd never felt as compatible with someone nor wanted anyone more than that person. And on the other hand, the slightly toxic dynamics of that relationship created more damage than I was willing to admit. Looking back, I think about the power of the chemistry and intensity of that relationship with a more clinical eye.

I've been in committed relationships that lasted years and had less impact. Yet, in that short relationship, I gave myself fully, rendered myself more open and vulnerable, all without the security of a reciprocal commitment. In the wake of that relationship, when I was finally ready to admit some serious healing had to begin, I decided to utilize all my psychotherapeutic knowledge to forge this pain into something new. And that's why I started my kundalini experiment.

As I stated in the introduction to this book, this approach is not for everyone. At that point in my life, I knew I was capable of handling such extremes, and decided I wanted to see what would happen if I could manage feeling everything all at once, and whether I would then be able to get to the bottom of it all. It wasn't easy. I became moody, irritable, and as the waves of emotions washed over me, I cried a lot. Deciding it wasn't productive, I resolved to calm down by meditating for hours at a time. When I finally found stillness, constructive thoughts started to come in, so I journaled quite a lot.

It's easy to get hung up on obsessive thoughts, going over and over the relationship in your mind, rehashing conversations and situations from the past, and not knowing how to stop those cyclical thoughts which are counter-productive to healing.

It's important to perceive such reflections as what they are—signs of anxiety dysfunctionally demonstrating that there's energy in your body you need to listen to and learn from. When you listen, you can write them down and treat those anxieties with empathy. Remember, these voices are a part of you. So the first part of calming them is listening to them and making them feel heard. In order to do this, you need to first be calm in order to calm those other parts of yourself. So before you sit down and to listening, perform your breathing exercises, and be your own source of stillness and strength. Only then can you hear what those voices have to say with the awareness required to provide you with what you need.

Attachment Hooks

One of the most difficult parts of moving on is holding onto the belief that this person is necessary for something. Let's start with examining what they provided. Was it something you never had before? For example, let's say they introduced you to a perspective, a different way of looking at yourself, or what you are worth. Just because it was new, and that person was the one who introduced that something new to you, that doesn't mean they are the only person who can give this to you. In fact, now that you know about it, it is there forever, and it is something that you can give to yourself.

If you believe that, you need a relationship to be okay, that's the first problem. Start by digging deep and uncovering your attachment hook. In the case of my 4 month relationship with the person I thought of at the time as the love of my life, it took me a while to figure it out that it wasn't him, but the lifestyle he had. He lived according to a very healthy routine. When we were together, I adopted those as my own, and living that routine together created a deep connection.

We were both focused on our health, which inspired intellectual conversations centered on expanding our mental and physical health. This felt like we were growing together and was something unique which I'd not experienced before. When I identified that as my attachment hook, I strengthened my routine, maintaining and enhancing it outside of that relationship. Since then, I've connected with people who live a similar lifestyle which I find attractive. I'm no longer hung up on any one person. Since my kundalini awakening, I've expanded my social circles, I'm making more friends than ever, and finding mentors who filled a void I didn't know was there. Not only are multiple individuals fulfilling my needs, but I found freedom, and this is a relationship of growth with myself.

However, it's important to recognize one of the more difficult attachment hooks to navigate are sexual, or even simple physical touch needs. This is something I often hear from my clients. "Other types of relations are not the same as a romantic connection." Yes, they are sexual and more touch-orientated in nature. However, that doesn't mean that you can't fulfill those needs yourself.

If you rely on others to fulfill those needs, you create dependency. As a sex therapist, I promote self-exploration as an activity that is as valuable as partner sex. Even though that's true, for many, on a scale from one to ten, masturbation can often come in at a level two, and exciting sex with a compatible partner can reach a level ten. Through meditation, breathwork, and other health practices, combined with self-exploration and understanding, you can achieve greater pleasure just by yourself. Yet, personally speaking, abstaining from partner sex, and giving myself time alone allowed me to discover partner sex wasn't necessary to my survival. There is a big difference between wanting and craving. Urges and cravings can sometimes lead us to unwanted situations and regretful actions. When you remove the animalistic value from your cravings, you are mindful of how to engage in the pleasures of the body.

In Kundalini, there are seven chakras that are in line with the spine. Each chakra are energy center that is considered Divine openings when they are unblocked and awakened. The sacral area is the second chakra, which is located in the lower abdomen, between your naval and pubic bone. This chakra is associated with sexuality, pleasure, connection, emotion, and creativity.

There are many things that can contribute to these blockages—trauma, pent-up emotions, residual past life issues, ancestral echoes—the stories of which don't even belong to you. So, the more mindful I was in my meditations, the more was able to successfully release these blockages from my sacral area, which were stored there from past generations, and other spiritual incarnations. Once I unblocked and awakened this chakra, I was able to enhance the pleasure I received in my genitals during masturbation, extending those feelings through to the rest of my body. I then no longer craved from men what I could achieve on my own, and was no longer dependent on partner sex.

So, when you find yourself cycling back to those feelings of loss, meditate on and define that attachment hook. Perhaps that person had a big personality that made you laugh and evoked a side of you no one has evoked before. Perhaps they activated a passion you haven't experienced before. Maybe they offered hope for the life, or a child, that you wanted. Identifying your unique hook is key to finding the right healing direction.

For example, if that person gave you pleasure, excitement, and passion, and you enjoyed their big energy, reclaim what they invoked within you as your own. Harness that energy within you and express that side of your personality without them. Identify what it was that stirred that passion and play with it. Find those feelings they shined a light on within you and cultivate that. Incorporate it into your life, explore it, and explore further. Do this and you'll very quickly find that you are no longer hooked on them. Remember, you were always the sole provider of that feeling. Only you can excite what is within you.

We don't really miss people; we miss what they invoked within us. All they did was help reveal that you needed more natural energy in your life. Although there are many energies a person can feel, that energy is not entirely unique and is not locked in a particular person. And that energy was within you all along, and it is still there. So, remember, often it isn't the person we miss, but how we relied on their energy to provoke those feelings within us. But instead of living in the absence of that energy, explore ways of evoking that energy, which was yours all along.

Here are a couple of exercises to intuitively understand what the emotional voices within you are saying, the hidden meanings behind your unhealthy thoughts, and how to make those emotional voices feel heard, understood, validated, comforted, and healed.

EXERCISE 6
Invoking Serenity

When you find yourself brooding and engaged in negative thoughts, write those thoughts down, one by one. Perform 10-15 minutes of breathing exercise. It can be as simple as counting 4 seconds for a breath-in and 4 seconds for a breath-out. I personally like to imagine a white, warm, healing light when I breathe in and a dark ash of negativity and anxiousness when I breathe out. When you do that, gently let your thoughts and emotions flow in for a brief moment, then capture them in a bubble which you will send floating away from you.

If feelings of sadness, anxiety, or loss start to rise when you attempt to let them go, return to focusing on your breath in between each bubble, and this will help you release those attachments. You need to un-anchor those clingy, self-afflicting thoughts. Instead, think about what those emotions are communicating, and that part within you that is voicing those emotions. Let that part know that you can give them what they need, and waste no time gently shifting your attention back to your breath.

If, however, you are still feeling distressed, continue your breathing exercises, or engage in other activities, you find calming and healthy and tap into the logical and rational parts of your mind. Once you feel you've calmed those rippling waters, write down some positive affirmations next to each of those negative ruminations. Soon, your inner dialogue will come to life.

Negative Rumination: "I'm so stupid, I should've known better!"

Affirmations: I'm not stupid (mention some good things that you've done in your life); I'm only human and humans make mistakes; I forgive myself for any actions I performed that were not in line with my values.

Reflection

If possible, at this stage, if you have been demonizing your ex, meditate on that for a moment. At this point, it's important to allow yourself to feel objectivity and let go of all judgment. Even if they were a bad person, you can give yourself permission to miss them. Just as you can give yourself permission to process your anger towards them if they were a good person. These are the most common emotions you need to process when it comes to a breakup, feelings of anger, and feelings of sadness or loss.

It's important to be objective. It's common to feel upset and to want to assign blame. Yet, this often prevents growth and recognizing how we contributed to the problems in that relationship. If, however, you find yourself glorifying your ex and can't seem to get over the fact that you're not together, it would serve you well to identify some realistic flaws they exhibited, problems that they brought into the relationship, those areas of incompatibility, and to objectify how they contributed to the breakup.

Putting them on a pedestal and blaming yourself is not being kind to yourself. When this is the case, the only relationship you should be focusing on is your relationship with you.

EXERCISE 7
Looking Forward

Anytime unwelcome negative ruminations arise, recognize them and perform the exercise above. Take a break and focus on calming your body and your mind. If you find those anxieties keep flooding in, try to calm yourself in other healthy ways. Reflect on a time where you independently felt good about yourself. Many of my clients often mention traveling, looking after a loved one, or taking on some fulfilling responsibilities as examples. Whatever yours is, tap into that calm state of mind before you address that inner voice, question it, and search for a deeper meaning behind it.

For example: "What a coward! They didn't even want to try working on our relationship!"

What are the unlying emotions there? Perhaps a fear of loneliness, pain of rejection, or feelings of inadequacy. You want to discover what those voices are really saying, what they might be deflecting, their motives, and identify those dysfunctional communication techniques.

In the statement above, we can see that here the speaker used blame and externalization. So, we are sending negative emotions outwards.

Questions to ask are:

"What if I didn't blame them? What would happen to me internally if it wasn't able to assign blame?"

"What does is this blame communicating to me? What is behind it?"

Too often, these negative thoughts center around feelings of worth. This exercise is intended to get you to start directly addressing your pain, which will better help you identify your attachment hooks. The more you approach this with curiosity and serenity, the more you'll be able to go beyond your ex-partner and understand the bigger story that has more to do with you.

During every difficult situation, we learn something new about ourselves and even this can trigger anxiety. This is especially true when avoid examining ourselves and project blame at the other party. Yet we cannot control our ex-partners, and that blame has little impact on their actions. So, the only things within our control are our attitudes, perception, and actions.

Such obsessive cyclical thoughts run over and over in our minds trying to show us where is the problem is, which often leads back to some early developmental wound or childhood trauma. In fact, we often gravitate towards partners that in some way help replay our childhood traumas or fears in an attempt to fix them.

For example, one of my childhood fears was a fear of abandonment. As a result, I often found myself with men who wanted me more than I wanted them, which made me feel more secure. Yet, what finally broke this pattern and moved past my fears was when I leaned into a relationship with someone who I truly wanted. Then, I actualized my fears when this relationship didn't work out. Giving my all to a relationship with someone who ended up being avoidant ironically helped me break my unhealthy, risk-avoidant pattern that was holding me back. This is a perfect example of how dormant trauma from the past can lure us into dysfunctional relationships. Only after that trauma is activated can it be healed. This is where the poison is also the antidote. I needed a dose of my own medicine to heal this wound that I didn't even realise existed.

The lesson I leaned at the end of it all was not to expect or demand love, not to take things personally, and to give more love to myself rather than hyper-focusing on whatever relationship I am in. Eventually, I reached a state of acceptance and self-compassion that overshadowed any sense of blame, victimization, or feelings of loss. And, when this is the case, it's important to be at peace with where you are, and remember how far you've come.

Personally, since I put in the work, I've realized that I now quickly outgrow my partners. When we first met, it seemed like we were at the same level, but in nearly every scenario, I outpaced them. So, rather than letting them hold me back, I decided I could hold space for them and wait for them to catch up. Call it a blessing and a curse. But I am prioritising myself and allowing myself to be close. It's okay to love intensely and then to move on. It simply means you have a great deal of energy, and are good at channeling that energy into yourself and healthy habits once that relationship is behind you. That energy can easily be channeled into beautiful things that you enjoy and are passionate about, such as creative pursuits and hobbies. Allowing yourself to be this way is rare, yes, but is something most people don't allow themselves to practice and yet envy in others. Simply permitting yourself to live this way, without guilt or shame, will better help you to heal and move on.

There is no shame in being different. It's also okay to be on a different vibrational level than someone else, whether lower or higher. Now, some people place judgment on someone with "lower" or "higher" vibrations. Yet, they are just vibrations. No, I aspire to reach the highest vibrational state I can in this lifetime, but I still acknowledge that being in a lower vibrational state merely means I am in a different classroom. Every soul has to go through each and every lesson at their own pace, and there is no skipping ahead.

I believe I have been through multiple horrible and volatile incarnations to finally reach where I am on my spiritual path. Just because a particular person doesn't match you energetically or practically is crucial when it comes to processing our feelings and permitting ourselves to detach quicker. When I first paired up with my Reiki practitioner Alex, he had issues going on in his life, and I found it difficult at times to be around him when his Kundalini Energy was so big it was contagious and affected me physically anytime I was around him.

It's difficult to commit to someone that is not on your same energetic level. But what if you were less energetic than your ex? If you weren't able to hold their energy, that's okay, too. Examine why you were in the relationship with them, and be honest with how it benefited you, and whether you can or cannot hold space for them.

Remember, we often end up attracting people who are on the same vibrational level, or who carry the same trauma in their bodies. Someone on a similar vibrational level is more likely to grow at your pace. Having energetic compatibility means being able to hold space for each other emotionally. And, at our core, we all want connection and understanding.

We've all had intense crushes with a self-awareness that they'll never evolve into anything, understanding that an infatuation doesn't need to equate to a soulmate. Along these lines, early on, I came up with practical reasons why I couldn't be with someone I was infatuated with. These were earthly reasons for deciding why I couldn't be in a prospective relationship with that crush. Reasons such as the feeling not being reciprocal, or such a relationship wasn't feasible because of professional boundaries, or because they lived in a different country. Yet, the animalistic part of me didn't pay much regard to these practical earthly reasons, and I still lusted after them.

So, that's when I decided I needed to pair earthly and practical as sharing spiritual reasons with each other. This perspective changed things. The moment I understood that a person couldn't hold me energetically and emotionally, I lost interest. So, I quickly found myself looking deeper into people's souls instead of only thinking of them in a practical sense. A connected relationship requires practical compatibility, such as sharing similar values and priorities, being on the same vibrational level, and sharing an image of the future.

This is a very different perspective than being in victim mode, when we reduce ourselves to nothing more than something insignificant that is pushed around by forces beyond our control, at the mercy of the storm. In victim mode we just sit there and do nothing, helplessly thinking, "what can I do?" But in truth, we are none of us insignificant. We are the storm. And, holding onto that perspective, finding balance within, you'll find it is your choice alone to allow something to sway you. Keep doing the work, and you'll find time truly does heal.

Chapter Five: Don't Overstimulate with Fixes – keep your mind on the game

Cyclical thoughts run the risk of becoming habituated, where nothing is accomplished, only fixating on what went wrong, what could have been done differently, while trying to redefine and justify our actions, and fix or repair the narrative of our pasts. Too often, such obsessive and negative ruminations result in a flood of self-afflicting emotions, such as anger or despair. And, as we covered earlier, emotional pain manifests physically, impacting the varying systems and structures of the body.

In such times of crisis, we tend to self-medicate. We submit to our cravings for escape, such as comforting ourselves through food, drugs, alcohol, overstimulation, avoidance, or risky sexual behavior. We're looking for a dopamine release, for feelings of euphoria, or a numbing of the pain. Therefore, neglecting such unprocessed emotions prolongs the damage to your psyche, increases obsessive thoughts, and delays healing. And it all begins again.

Look back at your life, and those moments you are not proud of or have come to regret. Now, imagine adding to them. A refusal to self-examine, to grow, and to incorporate those truths into your reality will only result in them sneaking back into your life in other toxic ways. For example, just like cyclical thoughts keep repeating over and over in your mind, those patterns will repeat in life. You'll end up in a similar relationship, repeating all the same mistakes and the same patterns. This is fairly universal, and we can all relate.

Recalibrating Your Focus and Intention

When our self-esteem is destabilised, it requires a great deal of energy to reinforce it. This goes beyond self-image. It requires establishing new habits, how we live our life, and our worldview. So, whether we care to admit it or not, relationships—even toxic ones—provide us with insight and self-awareness to process and build from.

However, the more independent and comfortable we get with being single, the greater the hesitation to surrender to a committed relationship, to vulnerability and open trust, with all its anxiety and uncertainty. Yet, in conflict with this, there is a fear of being alone! In order to navigate these overwhelming and confusing emotions, we need to learn how to connect and communicate better.

The Push and Pull of a Trauma Bond

As an only child with reliable and attentive parents, I feared losing the grounding stability they offered me, and feared being alone or on my own. I had no idea that these childhood fears would follow me well into adulthood. Counterintuitive to those insecurities, I consider myself to be fiercely independent—a side effect of being an only child. I traveled the globe by myself for three years, all while running my company, and I wasn't the type of person who would settle for just any relationship. So, I'd often opt for transitional relationships with a nice guy with whom I had little in common.

Having the upper hand in a relationship offered me a sense of safety, security, and superiority, where my armour couldn't be penetrated, and I could hold the emotional upper hand. Yet, in reality, this more so indicated a fear of being rejected by someone I wanted and who could penetrate my defenses. This had less to do with them, and more to do with trusting myself to do the work.

I wasn't ready to trust and to render myself vulnerable. It felt safer to keep the person I was with at a distance, and to *push* them away when

I needed. Predictably, a special someone came along, matching what I thought I wanted in my life, the type of person I hoped I could lean on and rely upon. This triggered a *pull*, which flooded in with intense feelings I didn't yet fully understand.

We commonly have a magnetic *pull*—or chemistry—with those who carry similar trauma as our own and therefore offer emotional compatibility. This is what I call a *trauma bond*. The more unresolved feelings you have, the greater the trauma bond. The stronger the chemistry, the harder it is to sort and process the chaos of those whirlwind emotions.

It wasn't until I found someone who I could open myself up to, and allow myself to be vulnerable with, did I experience the fear of losing them. I thought of myself as independent, not realizing I was capable of having intense and strong feelings for another until I met a partner who stirred those feelings within me. But I hadn't done the work, so didn't understand this at the time. And it wasn't until then that childhood fear rose to the surface. Such contradictions are more common than I'd taken for granted. The more you rely on a *trauma-bond* to offer you validation, or to fix your insecurities, the more work you need to put into yourself and into the relationship. But such a bond should never serve as a substitute for putting in the work. When neglecting to tend to wounds, they'll fester. When you haven't done the work, the more troubled the relationship becomes. And when the relationship ends, such a breakup will become that much harder to move on from, reopening old wounds, all the way back to childhood. This inevitably results in that much more work which needs to be done than before.

The more self-aware you are of your feelings, the less likely you are to repeat unhealthy patterns in your relationships. So, it's important to recognize and label those dysfunctional coping strategies people most commonly turn to. I call such distractions "fixes". A lot of things can be used as a fix. Some are easily identifiable, such as an increase in alcohol intake, binge-eating, smoking, irritability, and excessive shopping.

So, here is a list of *fixes* that may not be universally obvious. With each example, I'll offer suggestions on how to shift a fix from something unhealthy into a fulfilling part of your life.

PHYSICAL EXERCISE

As much as I highly recommend exercise, it's important to recognize when you are approaching it from an unhealthy mindset. For many, when they exit a relationship, it's common to turn to exercise, hoping to fix their self-image. We all want to feel and look more attractive in hopes of attracting a potential partner. But this should be approached for the right reasons and with a healthy mindset, as opposed to being motivated by feelings of self-blame, shame, fear, or trying to meet the other's expectations or seeking external validation.

When addressing this fix, you don't necessarily need to decrease the amount of exercise you perform; you just need to adjust the way you approach it. Imagine a woman who exited a relationship with a partner that she exercised with quite often. Then, after the relationship, she felt she needed to meet a specific standard and needed external validation to feel attractive and appealing to men. So, when she gets attention at the gym, it promotes her self-esteem. Yet, the novelty of this soon wears off.

Eventually, she loses motivation and starts listening to music while exercising. Soon that's not enough, and she's watching TV, always needing more stimulation to keep going. Yet, in the end, she realises she didn't like exercising all that much and was only doing it for validation. So, her motivation was 60% fighting her insecurities and only 40% motivated by improving her health.

Now, in contrast, imagine that same woman taking an entirely different approach to exercise altogether. She instead starts going out into nature with no other external stimulation or validation required. The more she listened to her body, the more she realised it was speaking back to her. The more mindful she was, the more she enjoyed it, and the more self-love she was able to express through her intentions. The self-love manifests in the form of calm positivity, a more centered and balanced emotional state, which she shares with the world through her every interaction. That calm positivity has a physical impact on everyone who encounters her energy.

Emotional growth is connected to body growth. The more positivity you make space for in your body, the more room you make for healing, moving different parts of your body in the right direction. This can lead to physical and mental changes, to euphoria, negative energy leaving your body, and feelings of elation and weightlessness. The dark clouds above you will clear. You'll be more in tune with the healthy voices within you, listening when your body tells you to train more and to rest.

Getting into such a mindful practice takes work. This is something I myself often struggled with. You see, I have a practical mind, which can sometimes cause me to impatiently leap ahead, skipping important steps such as properly warming up. However, doing this demonstrated a lack of commitment. Something that is viewed as a means to an end is not something that is treated with love. When I eventually approached exercise with more mindfulness, I experienced better results with the same exercises and equipment than I had before. I also found I was releasing more emotional trauma from my body at a faster rate.

My whole life I hated cardio and running. But as soon as I learned to perform cardio, in balance with strength training, I was better able to monitor my emotions and self-soothe. I was healing both physically and psychically. Self-conscious and self-deprecating thoughts were soon replaced with self-reassurance and self-love. In no time, as soon as I started exercising for all the right reasons—primarily for all of myself—I saw results that always evaded me otherwise. To this day, when I exercise, I never feel alone. I often imagine that I'm running (or doing other things) with a silhouette of me that is there to constantly support me. I even joined an awesome gym called the Temple of Mastery, through which I've met an amazing community of like-minded people.

In the past, I resisted spending money on gym memberships. Yet, as you change, your priorities change as well. It provides an amazing emotional release and I can't fathom not having it in my life. It helps me to test myself, to work on my emotional regulation, and I get cranky if I can't move my body enough in a week. I pay attention to those voices within me, which communicate in varying ways. Such as when I start to feel insecure while I'm running, I'm more prone to getting stitches in my side. I also train when my body tells me to, and I regularly enjoy cardio and yoga.

So, absolutely exercise and focus on your emotional and physical health! But think about how you approach it. Are you using this as a fix, and what is the motivation behind it, and what are you trying to fix? Are you trying to heal and do the work and improve yourself? Or are you doing it to escape, or to gain the approval of others? The more mindful of your reasons and your emotions, the more you'll be able to move past the breakup and move forward for yourself.

MUSIC

Music makes us feel good, and it's easy to get lost in it. But I need you to ask yourself whether you are using music as a fix. Are you escaping into music to avoid doing the work? Answer honestly, and if any of your inner voices say yes, before any of those other inner voices have the chance to talk over that *yes*, then it's time to shift your intention. You don't have to give up music. You just have to reclaim it.

David Goggins, a famous athlete and motivational speaker, once said, "Listening to music during training is cheating." It is indeed a very pleasurable thing to do, but if you're drawing energy from the music, rather than from the activity itself, you are not training your body and mind in the same capacity. Music can boost your sports performance, numb or validate the pain, and silence unwelcome thoughts from coming in. So, again, we need to recalibrate your focus and intention. The same principle applies to music as it does to exercise. If you want to purely enjoy it for itself, don't do anything else when you are listening to it. Be mindful of your body and the way it's feeling. Experience that music for the love that you feel for it, for yourself and how it makes you feel, and for those who you want to share it with.

Doing one activity at a time helps train your mind, refocus your intention, and to grow in a way that enables you to quickly outgrow the relationship you are leaving behind. When you outgrow the relationship, you no longer long for it. It becomes easier to recognise that stress and longing as undesirable self-afflicting emotions. And, once you no longer use it as a fix, there's nothing wrong with listening to music with intention, even when it is on in the background or when you exercise at the gym. Just pay attention to your intentions.

When you live with someone, it is common over time to develop a heightened sense of empathy or experiencing some level of empathic mirroring. This is where you experience some level of another person's emotional or physical state. Although this isn't universally experienced, to different degrees, it is more common than not. After my Kundalini awakening, my empathy heightened, to the point where I experienced others' energies and feelings with greater intensity. I felt highly intuitive about whether the feelings I was picking up on were coming from a male or female, often tuned into what was afflicting them. So, I often use music to help me stay centred in my world, instead of taking in other people's unwelcome emotions. Focussing on those intentions can be very useful when trying to avoid co-dependencies.

I also like to listen to music to ignite feelings that I've found more difficult to work through in a positive way. For example, I sometimes test myself by listening to songs that remind me of my ex. I call this practice *reclaiming*. When untangling the music from the *ex-association*, at some point, those emotions fade and the song is *reclaimed*. This is another method of refocusing your intentions regarding a fix. You can practice the same thing with places where you frequented with your ex. Spend time alone in that place while writing in your journal, or meditating and breathing through those difficult feelings while enjoying your own company.

Performing reclaiming activities is useful for anything you want disassociated from an ex, be it a word, a sentence, or objects that remind you of them. Every time you stumble upon an association with that relationship, take it as an opportunity to work through those feelings. Every fix needs an intention. That's when it stops being a fix. But first, you need to understand how any particular activity became a fix in the first place. This requires an honest dialogue with your inner voices, and what the different parts of you are trying to communicate. What are the emotions behind those behaviours? Once you understand this, you can easily refocus your intentions and enjoy every pleasurable activity for what it offers, rather than what it doesn't.

SOCIAL INTERACTION

It's natural right after a breakup to look to others for the much-needed validation that is absent once a relationship is ended. So, we reach out to those who we can rely upon. We reach out to our best friends, our family, our siblings. But there is a danger of habitualising this as well, becoming dependent on them, with a constant need for external validation and assurance that everything will be all right, or that we are good enough to carry on. This is a clear sign one hasn't fully carried on.

We all need a sympathetic ear from time to time, especially when we're feeling emotional or our sensitivity is heightened. But this should only serve as a temporary fix. If you get in the habit of expecting others to take on your emotional load for you, you won't learn to deal with it yourself. At some point, preferably early on, we need to pick ourselves up and be self-reliant enough to embark on performing the work primarily on our own.

The best method for tracking your progress is by practicing being mindful of how much you feel the need for this external unburdening. If your conversations feel repetitive, and you feel like you are spinning your wheels, you are most likely locked in a cycle of pain. When this is the case, refocus your intention. What does expressing what you are experiencing offer? Are you hoping that their reassurances and expressions of affection will fix you? Or are you taking advantage of the rewarding qualities of the relationship you have with that person, actually listening to their advice, and doing the work of sorting through your emotions by verbally expressing them? If you feel calmer, gain new helpful insights about yourself and your relationship, and process your feelings of anger and loss, you can give yourself a pat on the back. If not, then you might consider interacting with others in a more useful way.

Practice being more mindful about your intentions during a conversation. For example, if you feel the urge to complain or lecture someone, question whether this is a fix instead of a genuine connection. Or, if you feel you are seeking someone's approval, this is also an indicator that you are looking for a fix. The way to recognize a social interaction fix is by being honest about your expectations of others.

Start by spending more time listening to others, and giving freely rather than wielding expectations or going in with ulterior motives. Be more mindful of your emotions, what your body is telling you, and of what you want to say. Doing so will help you better refocus your intentions and mindfulness. When you do participate in conversations, make sure your remarks reflect your values. Monitor how much of your emotional load you share—limit it to a reasonable amount—and enquire about their emotional world.

It's important during such times that you nurture your relationships rather than overburden them. This type of mindful communication will enrich your relationships and will promote true connection that can help mitigate the loss of a relationship and promote true healing. Focus your intentions on the joy those social interactions offer, rather than using them as an outlet for your emotional load. Doing that will only promote discord in the relationship. Rather, nurture those relationships, and enjoy what they have to offer. Of course, you'll end up talking about what you are going through and experiencing. And there is nothing wrong with that as long as you focus on regulating your emotions and taking what that social interaction has to offer towards your healing.

It's common to feel as if your world suddenly got smaller and that feeling of loss that comes with the absence of an intimate partner. During such times, it's easy to forget that we have other important people in our lives. The nature of the permanence of life shows us any connections we create. They are never owned by us, and must be embraced without expectations but with calm boundaries which we set for ourselves. And when our hearts are distressed, it's not uncommon to take those reliable friendships for granted, especially when there is a void to fill.

As soon as you refocus your intentions and your energy and start shifting your priorities elsewhere, that void becomes smaller until it eventually disappears. This practice can be difficult at first. But, the more you mitigate how much of your energy you spend on self-serving emotional unburdening and mining for validation, the more you will find genuine fulfillment from those social interactions which promote genuine connection. One method is to practice a type of compassion which is separate from empathy.

Compassion communicates, "I care about your issues, but I don't make them my own." Whereas empathy, on the other hand, communicates, "I care about your issues so much that they also make me sad." Now, when refocusing these intentions, you have to be mindful to not make such social interactions transactional. Doing this right can be challenging, but the point is to focus on doing the work and healing rather than relying on a fix that gets you nowhere. So, what does this look like? Well, in your social interactions, this may require you to give more energy than you receive, which can prove challenging when your energy reserves are already running low. So the aim is to find balance without it becoming transactional. Giving to such relationships without expectations will be more fulfilling, allow for more genuine connection, greater balance, and participation in growth.

Now, there are certainly those who struggle with asking for help. If you are connection-avoidant, this could be a growth area from which you would likely benefit. Try leaning on those friends who are willing to be there for you, just as you are ready to be there for them. If doing so terrifies you or generates anxiety, go towards it and get acquainted with that until it stops scaring you. If this sounds like you, you're not alone, and these feelings are more common than you think.

If you find yourself paralysed, take a moment to go into silence and attentively listen to what your voices are telling you. Then decide which of those voices you want to voice as your own. Rather than adopting voices that scream out your insecurities which didn't exist before that relationship, put them there, reclaim your voice. After taking that moment, start small. Start engaging in social interactions with random people and acquaintances, which come with lower expectations. Then move into socialising with close friends.

Try not to worry about them, judging the scope of your strengths based on your vulnerabilities. Remember, they have their own journey to navigate. With most friendships, you are sharing a journey, walking side by side. So sharing is key. But there needs to be a balance. This means accepting people for who they are. There's no need to leave them behind, which, the more emotionally aware you are, is less likely a compulsion.

Leaning on family for some can prove most difficult, as was the case with me. There is so much history there, which can complicate things. In my Polish family, there is a notion that you *expect* to be loved no matter what happens and what you do. The problem is a true connection doesn't blossom in the presence of expectations. So, considering that as a cultural component, that leads to an expectation that you *deserve* to be loved and supported by family, no matter what. But, this is counter to doing the work. We can't demand or expect this from anyone; otherwise, it becomes a fix. Instead, the aim must be to ensure every connection is genuine and fulfilling.

SOCIAL MEDIA

It's generally accepted that decreasing the time spent on social media is correlated with improved mental health. Yet, despite the fact that there is a common perception that social media can be an unhealthy addiction, there can be ways of incorporating it into our daily routine safely. Most of us engage in it for our own reasons. It is, however, important to develop some internal boundaries to prevent it from becoming a habituated fix. It's important to recognize it can serve as an easy outlet for external validation. This is something that can easily be evaluated simply by paying attention to your previous posting habits.

However, this is yet another opportunity for self-betterment. Pay closer attention to how you feel when you spend time on social media. Refocus your intentions here as well and be more meditative in what you post. Try to avoid attention-calling, and instead post for the love of yourself and to support and show your love to others, business reasons are also valid. For example, when I post on social media these days, you'll find that my posts are typically practical, drawing attention to an event, or to something I found inspiring that I wanted to share, or some activity I wanted to share with friends and clients. I truly believe the intention behind it needs to be pure and self-centered.

It is absolutely important to recognize and embrace when you're feeling insecure. This way, when such feelings arise, you can respond to what your inner voices are asking of you. You can reassure yourself and perform an inner check-in. Especially if you find yourself experiencing feelings of insecurity, such as issues with not wanting to post pics of yourself.

Remember, allowing people to see you is also a form of courage and vulnerability. I'm not talking about posting revealing pictures or anything like that. However, it is important to overcome insecurities that might prevent you from posting a photo of you and your friends. Posting selfies and being proud of the way you look can also be refocused. You don't want to use this activity as a fix, where you are attention-seeking for external validation. Just be authentic in how you show yourself, and your intentions will become pure. I like to take nice photos of myself now and again and post them online. But, I try to approach it from the mindset of, "I love my body, and I'm not afraid to show it."

If you are spending an obsessive amount of time on social media, consider decreasing it. Our bodies are not accustomed to that much dopamine being released from these deliberately addictive algorithms and the supply-trained behavioral rewards from videos and images. So, if you need to decrease your time on social media, you can try using your phone only during certain times of the day. You can even use an automated lockbox and put your phone there while you are doing other things.

I believe social media can be a great way to speak your truth and practice showing your true self to the world while maintaining a record of your journey. So, when dedicating time to such activities, refocus your intention and post a few times a week about your self-development journey to inspire others while showing yourself how far you've come.

READING BOOKS AND WATCHING MOVIES

We all take pleasure in escaping into a good book or a good movie. In fact, there is absolutely nothing wrong with this when the intention is focused. It's common to search for answers to your problems in books—such as this one! This is why it's important to put what you learn from them into practice and do the work. A self-help book is there to help you help yourself. But simply reading a book isn't the same experience as putting the self-help advice it offers into practice.

Mindful activities will train your brain and will develop a true love for those activities and balance your self-esteem. So, how to make sure that books and movies are not a fix, but add value to your life? How do you ensure this lovely activity is a way through which you can express some love to yourself? Again, using mindfulness and recognizing when you are siphoning the energy from the stories instead of just enjoying the read. Recognize your intention. If it's taking you away from your body and mind, you are most likely using it as an escape. But, if you can focus on your emotions and address them as they come up, while genuinely engaged in the story, you are doing it!

However, I am 100% guilty of a common fallacy here. It was all too easy for me to mask a lack of inner work by escaping into romance novels and rom-coms. These escapes sell a fantasy in the form of hope for future love. It provides an outlet for feeding off of, and living vicariously through others' experiences. It is absolutely an escape and a fix. Waiting for love is a problematic ideal built into society. It can even stand in the way of enjoying that love that we could experience instead of waiting for the Hollywood image of an intimate partner.

Think about the word *waiting*. This suggests living in scarcity. When you live with a scarcity mindset, what the universe offers will reinforce your mindset. So, what does that look like? Repeating the same patterns, finding yourself dating similar partners, and experiencing all the same problems as before. This is why I've made a practice of saying to myself—for the Universe to overhear—*I have everything I need and more, and I welcome new abundance into my life.*

If, after a breakup, spending time with family and friends, or spending time alone falls utterly short of spending time with that ex who is no longer in your life, then that relationship was likely transactional, and not unconditional. When you struggle with properly expressing your love with yourself, and with your family and friends, you'll likely find romantic love difficult to navigate. This is why it's important to go in without expectations, and allowing only good and healthy people in your life. This will create assuredly manifest more feelings of abundance and fulfillment in your life.

Now I have refocused my intentions when escaping into romantic novels and movies. Romantic love can be more complex and wields the promise of genuine connection. The more compassion I have for those characters, facing similar situations, the more I gather this compassion for myself. My emotions come to the surface when engaged in those stories. I cry, I relate, and I let go. This has also offered me a greater understanding of my obsession with historical movies.

I've carried massive amounts of transgenerational trauma in my body. I found ways of expressing that trauma by paying tribute to my ancestors through immersing myself in their stories, especially those reenactments which so accurately portrayed their lives. The body knows how to heal itself, and I approach watching war movies with that intention, making room to honor my ancestors and their pain.

TRAVELING

Imagine someone who longs to have the same experience as a great philosopher who uncovered incredible mysteries by going off and being a hermit. So, imagine this person, seeking that experience, does what they did, going into confinement in search of life's mysteries. Yet, over time this person misses their friends, their home, and after a year, returns home with little to show for that experience. Yet, could that have gone differently? What if they leaned into the discomfort of being alone, questioned what those friendships were providing, and tried to find ways to find in isolation what they gained from those friendships?

What does it mean to find yourself? What about you are you trying to tap into? What mystery are you trying to uncover? People say that you find yourself when you travel and this often can prove true. In some ways, it was true for me. When I spent three years traveling across over 30 countries, I tested myself, and I grew a lot. I mostly traveled solo and had the freedom to come and go as I pleased. It was the time of my life, and an experience I'll never regret. I felt free, and not burdened by other people. Nevertheless, I realize that this too was an escape.

I didn't necessarily mind traveling with someone, but I perceived it sometimes as a bit of a burden. However, there are many out there who only travel with friends because they love being around people, giving and receiving connection, and people-pleasing to ensure that dynamic. Even though there is a difference between the reasons behind traveling with others and traveling alone, both versions can be a fix.

The more I grew, I started recognizing that backpacking wasn't as enticing as it used to be. As I grew and found more compassion for myself, I was drawn to healthier activities. Not to say the activity of backpacking isn't healthy. Rather, it was the lifestyle that came with it, that of living in dorms and staying in hostels. The socializing and drinking were not healthy nor facilitated growth. Now, I traveled this way for a long time, and bear no judgment to those who enjoy it. It served as part of my journey to self-betterment.

We need to experience those journeys to determine what matters most in our lives. I also realized that I got a kick out of having *checked off* more and more places, thinking I would seem *cooler* for the more places I'd been. But that approach led to me rushing through some of those experiences, and thereby experiencing them less. This was an exhibition, not an experience. It was me saying, look where I've been.

So, travel with mindfulness. Slow down and experience it for all the right reasons. Let it help you grow in unpredictable ways. Think about what you want to do when you're there, instead of what others are doing. And, if you find you aren't experiencing the experience of travel, and only thinking of getting back home, or where you are heading next, as yourself why you are there, and what you are running from.

CLEANING

Since childhood, I have had issues keeping my space clean. I resisted cleaning and tidying my space, even in adulthood, out of practical reasons. It didn't make sense to make my bed when I was just going to mess it up again. My mom, on the other hand, always kept things pristine, and is still quite particular about how things should be cleaned. Both of us were approaching cleaning in the wrong way. For her, it was something that she could control and a way to express empathy for others and the space. I was exhibiting self-serving behavior and didn't find cleaning practical.

However, my mother used to always relay the adage, *"Your personal space is a reflection of who you are."* I understand this now on a deeper level. Countless studies have revealed that having a clean and orderly personal space reduces stress and anxiety, offers a sense of control, and reduces visual overstimulation—when your space is disorderly and chaotic, it can bombard your senses and overwhelm you emotionally. (Brass 2019, p. 22) Also, it can promote better sleep, enhance your mood, boost mental clarity, focus, and offer you with a more peaceful and meditative safe space.

Today, I wouldn't say I've entirely changed. But my intentions are refocused. When I clean, or choose not to clean, I don't do so for practical reasons or for others. I make those choices because it's something I choose to do for my own mental health, and for love of myself and for others. I don't obsessively clean up every single time, but I also mostly keep on top of it so it doesn't pile up at the end of the week, and result in overstimulation.

MEDITATION AND MINDFUL ACTIVITIES

Up to this point, I've been an advocate for practicing mindfulness. Yes, and I still absolutely do. Nevertheless, it is at this juncture that I need to warn against overdoing it. It is also worth confessing that at one time, when I was at a low point, I used this as a fix. I even convinced myself doing so would *fix* all my emotions and pain. What I didn't realise at the time, though, was that if you meditate for too long, you can induce anxiety, increasing your cortisol levels, as a result of becoming too aware of yourself and the world too quickly.

Similar to traveling, when you are meditating, you are exploring your consciousness. Meditating to too great an excess won't allow you to experience and integrate all the knowledge about yourself and the world that is being revealed to you. You can't rush through it and experience it. Mindfulness cannot be rushed and must be practiced. So, it's important to make time for *Earthly* things, like going to the shops, seeing friends, and other material pursuits. You need to afford your life the ability to catch up with your spiritual development, otherwise you might experience derealization or depersonalization. I refer to it as being trapped in between dimensions. So, make sure you take time to recenter yourself, to be *right here and right now*, while monitoring your thoughts and feelings.

Your Inner Power

This chapter has worked up to separating fixes from escapes. We need those moments where we can shut off our brains and empty our heads. An escape, like a good book, going to the gym, socializing, or spending time on social media can be a necessary reward at the end of a day, as long as you are not using that escape as a means of avoiding doing the work, or a false fix to your problems. And escape, when indulged in mindfully, can provide that necessary dopamine release, helping you recharge, and contributing to your *inner power*. You, standing on your own, without most of your fixes, embody the truest version of *you* that you can find!

Enjoying those activities mindfully can provide an escape, especially when we are mindful about what those experiences truly have to offer. But, the second they are misused, and that fix is habituated for the wrong reasons as a fix, that's when it becomes a problem. But enjoying such activities from time to time, while making space for acknowledging your feelings as you perform these activities, creates balance. You enjoy it more, and it becomes a healthy coping strategy.

Habitualise a fix, and taking it too far, will overstimulate your brain, which will lead to producing less natural dopamine, thereby compromising your inner power. When you overdo it, you're blind to where the pain is coming from, making it harder to refocus your intentions and harder for you to heal.

I often hear my clients say, *"I just need to shut off my mind."* You can take two dramatically different paths when it comes to *shutting off*. The first one is via a *numbing* and *fixing* activity, and is temporary and unsustainable. The other option is training your mind to become *calmer* and *easier to navigate*. If you must engage in your fixes for a short period as a means of damage control, by all means. But as you engage in your fixes, bear in mind what is actually happening. Be mindful at all times, otherwise you'll be at risk of a dependency on that fix, and it will end up being harder to come back from. A balance between your fixes, mindfulness, and self-reassurance is the key to establishing a good routine.

EXERCISE 8
Fix to Healthy Coping Strategy

It's impossible to live life without our fixes. So, we need to choose those that will add the most value to our lives. With the right mindful practice,

they can be healthy or useful coping strategies. So, start by making a list of all the fixes or escapes you lean on. Here are a few examples:
- Exercising (cardio and strength training)
- Stretching/ yoga
- Mindful and grounding practices
- Seeing friends and venting (sometimes)
- Joking (also to laugh at the pain very often)
- Eating healthy (the 80/20 principle-eating healthy 80% of the time and 20% is for fun)
- Scrolling on social media (just a few minutes a day)
- Going out to see events
- Not watching my posture when I'm tired
- Having the heater all night turned on (I can't stand the cold)
- Netflix
- Buying new clothes not for practical reasons
- Taking a long shower
- Wearing something that makes me feel confident

Next, in a state of reflection, while being mindful and refocusing your intentions with each activity, strategize how you can use all of your small fixes to help you on this journey without overusing any one of them. The goal is to alternate between them, changing their intentions from being a fix to healthy coping strategies. You want to keep them balanced and plan out how you can realistically create new routines where they fit into the growth you are seeking in your life, which, in turn, will facilitate healing. This practice will keep you from putting all of your eggs in one basket and creating a codependent relationship with the part of your life you are trying to let go of.

Clarify Retrospection

As we know, the stress hormone cortisol can damage our physiology. However, it can also heal it. This is why it's considered normal to lean towards extremes after going through some sort of psychological trauma and internal chaos. We jump into extreme behaviors because we are wired to. Trauma seeks trauma, and each trauma triggers the body to heal itself. This presents a paradox.

Pain and endurance offer an opportunity for experiential learning. It offers the promise of making us stronger and more resilient to the pain we might create for ourselves in the future. This is how pursuing extremes often leads to a psychological or physically addictive fix. However, if you don't monitor the *destruction*, it can quickly become unmanageable. The challenge is to surrender to the pain, pay attention to it, and to learn from it. This is approached without betraying our boundaries, and in so doing, creates a more fluid growth transition without causing unmitigated damage.

It takes practice to permit our sufferings to destroy what they need to. Doing so creates room for us to pick up the pieces when we regain our strength later on. Think of it as simply allowing the past to move into the past, or as letting go of something that is already lost. This is simply a sad, yet necessary truth of life. Allow those ego attachments to fade, self-reflect, refocus, and look back on what that time symbolised for you with a clearer view.

Letting go is different from surrendering control to the trauma. Left to its own devices, the trauma will seek more trauma, enabling an endless chain of trauma-seeking behavior and avoidance through fixes, ultimately leading to self-destructive tendencies. This is what leads to binge drinking, seeking intimacy before you're ready, and any other distractions that lead to more problems. Having said this, it's important not to demonize your fixes. Rather, be gentle with yourself, and don't turn unhealthy habits into taboos. Doing so may run the risk of rebelling against convention and seeking out the self-destructive behaviors you are trying to mindfully refocus into healthier habits. It's all too easy to stray off in a direction that's not aligned with your values.

When you are not learning from your experiences, it's harder for the body and mind to heal. So start by paying attention to all the ways your emotions are manifesting, such as your posture, body temperature, and general health. Remember early on when we discussed *the child versus the adult brain*? The *adult brain* is often not available when we are in turmoil. So, recognising this, think of yourself as a kid that just needs a bit of love, nurturing, care, and help. What do children need? To feel safe. To feel loved and cared for. They need stability, routine, and someone to rely upon.

The more self-soothing you are, the more stability you'll implement for the person who needs it most: you. Think of it this way. When the most important person in your life needs you the most, you drop everything and selflessly come to their rescue. And the most important person in your life is you. Healing doesn't happen overnight. But centering yourself is crucial to the healing process. By centering, I mean a constant refocus on the now. To truly process and heal our pain, we first must allow ourselves to feel it. We need to pay attention to what our bodies are telling us, and to make all of our inner voices feel heard. If we don't, then all the different energy systems of our bodies and mind will be at conflict with one another, and they will each feel alone and become bitter, reckless, or stagnant.

The first and most difficult lesson is listening to those truths which are the hardest to hear. But with mindful practice, and through refocusing our intentions, we'll slowly build up the courage to listen, process, perform the work that needs to be done, which is more pleasurable over time.

Chapter Six: Don't Under Stimulate and Process Your Emotions

The days that lead up to a breakup can often bear the burden of a heightened intensity, which can send you into crisis mode. During these times, that intensity can easily be projected outward towards your friends, family, and those you console with and lean on. After a breakup, in these situations, it's common to reflect and feel like you have *been too much*, especially if you were the one that was broken up with. This frequently leads to the extreme of withdrawing, wanting to avoid your world seeing you at a low point.

When experiencing any sense of loss or mourning, it is difficult to put on a smile and pretend you are okay. Directing what little energy you have to put on a mask to avoid attracting attention to your feelings of vulnerability. Those who are prone to avoidance and withdrawal as a mechanism will need to be particularly careful to find the right balance, and in every scenario, balance needs to be a priority. When this is the case, you must be mindful of finding the space to soothe yourself, and the self-compassion to find safety in reaching out to friends and family.

Becoming a hermit and staying home and doing nothing is tempting. I've been there. However, it frequently puts us on a fast track to depression. Remember, stimulation deprivation and withdrawal can become a form of escape. This includes withdrawing from social engagements or avoiding any aspects of your life that may seem overwhelming. It often leads to hyper-focusing solely on your isolation and numbness, while avoiding everything else.

Even when that one activity is focusing on our healing, performing that one activity can also be destructive. For example, after isolating at home and overdoing it on my Kundalini meditations, I was forced to address my lack of balance. My hyper-focus and fixation led me down a pretty dangerous path. Not only did I run the risk of regressing, I wasn't moderating my meditation practices, and for a short period, experienced difficulty retaining fluids and solid food. This forced me out of isolation and to seek some help in restoring my balance so that I could finish the work.

We often don't realize it when we've been hyper-focusing either on the self or the external world. Both cases can be dangerous. I was so fixated on my experimental cure that I was neglecting the voices that the different energy systems of my body were communicating to me. As a result, I wasn't seeing clearly what needed my attention and those parts of me that needed healing the most.

Disasters Walk in Pairs

In Poland, we have a saying, "disasters walk in pairs." Meaning, we attract those who are on a similar wavelength. There are many fields of science that explore this reality. Some call it brainwaves, other explain it as relating to pheromones. Others discuss the vibrational levels in the body and we attract situations and people on the same vibrational level. Such as, after dating a narcissist, you are more likely to attract yet another, perhaps even worse narcissist, that can perhaps teach you a lesson that you need to be looking out for yourself first. But when you carry trauma within your body, you'll attract those with similar struggles and inner conflicts or perceptions. Quite often, this can lead to pairing up with someone who can add to that trauma and make their situation even worse.

For example, imagine a person who is coping with their trauma, yet their commitment is fragile. Then they meet someone with similar trauma, who is habitually reliant on their fixes, and racing down a path of self-destruction. Yet, they have chemistry and share a genuine connection. Next thing they know, they're both on the same path of self-destruction, sharing that trauma, transforming their fragile situation into a disaster. *Disasters walk in pairs.*

This sad story is all too common, and it rarely has a happy ending. Anytime we find ourselves in a low place, trouble has an easy time of working its way into our lives. This can contribute to the internal struggles of our urges and our subconscious mind, and will increase the likelihood of choosing worse and worse partners in the future. And when those internal struggles turn into inner conflict, or all out war between our different parts, it's a sign of those inner voices becoming angrier or more irrational.

There is nothing wrong with being emotionally demonstrative. But being self-aware is important, and without doing the work, how can you trust where those emotions are coming from? For example, is your emotional display coming from something you've been holding in? As you held it in, did more things get shoved in with it? Has the pressure been building? Do you find more and more little things frustrating you and making you angry? If the answer to these is yes, then you haven't been doing the work, and you've compromised your mental and physical health. You run the risk of becoming bitter, getting angrier over time, and becoming more explosive through their reactions. That frustration grows into anger, which only escalates.

What comes out in those outbursts isn't solely just frustration and anger, but the accumulated trauma that's been neglected. The way to break this pattern is to identify the trauma by listening to *all* of your inner voices and doing the work. The more focused you are on doing the work, the sooner you can put an end to it. Contrary to popular belief, you can change your temper. In fact, you can change your whole personality to serve you better in life. It's a lot of work, but it's absolutely worth it.

You can manifest your life and reality when you are in tune with yourself and others, learning to handle difficult emotions, while promoting mindful compassion.

Perform the work mindfully and on your own terms. This is within your control. The other path too often leads to damage and more trauma. And, if you leave your emotional world unattended to, a future partner found in desperation will, at some point, make you look into that emotional mirror, anyway. Wouldn't it be so much more fulfilling to look at it of your own accord, making those changes regardless of your life situation, *instead of letting trauma force you to look?*

Nearly everyone carries trauma in their bodies that they are either not aware of, or are intentionally not addressing. These can be childhood traumas, recent emotional wounds, and even generational traumas from members of our family, or even those in our family line that we've never met. And when you neglect that which demands your attention, this can lead to trouble.

Try to design your life in a way that you want to heal and to do the work. Your life will be much more fulfilling. If it's not, another emotional block will come up, which will introduce more trauma, and another missed opportunity to learn the lesson from it. Improving means analyzing your thoughts, feelings, and patterns, going through your childhood experiences, and making peace.

Many of your inner voices are resonances of childhood trauma, in which case you need to get your emotional *kindergarten* in order before it takes over and creates more trouble later on. This requires a commitment to healing and creating a psychologically healthy plan of action. You will need to stop and listen to what all the voices within you are saying. And in response to their impulses, their wants, and their needs, you need to guide them, offer them your wisdom, and parent them. Show those parts of you that you care deeply for them, and want the best for them as you go about your life.

This is how you can process your difficult feelings while enjoying your life. Give yourself permission to *feel*, to jump back and forth between joy and suffering. And when you suddenly have feelings of relief, don't try to banish them out of guilt or shame. Don't punish yourself for having a laugh. Anytime the burden is lifted, know that's your body's way of trying to heal itself. So give yourself permission to feel all of your emotions. Finding that balance is crucial. That's what life is, a constant change of the energy inside of you. We can't be always happy and we don't have to be always sad either. Provide space for both.

If you practice gratitude and self-compassion, even when it is difficult and your turbulent emotions present an obstacle to doing so, *what you promote will become your reality*. Everyone has something to work on. Learning how to calm down when you get angry or resentful, and analysing why you get like this in the first place will allow you to process those stored emotions that you have accumulated over the years. But remember that some emotions will not make sense, but we need to feel through them anyway without questioning them.

Whenever you start to reshape your reality and mould it to your desire, serendipity will present itself. New wonderful opportunities, friends, and experiences will come your way, and what you want for yourself will manifest. For some, it might feel like a self-fulfilled prophecy. For others, divine intervention. The important thing is to find meaning in it, and approach it with gratitude and compassion.

EXERCISE 9
Adult in the House

Being in practice of a mindful life is crucial for our personal growth. It's important to understand how susceptible you are to the influences of your different internal voices, and the level of control which you surrender to any one of them at any moment. This is why it is important to perform mindful check-ins several times a day, and at least twice a day as a beginning point. Keeping this in mind, you can apply this exercise at any point in time.

When starting your check-in, listen to your body and identify any tension, funny sensations, waves of emotion, anything that speaks out of you, try to be in tune with it. Identify which part of you is speaking to you right now and acknowledge it. Name it. If you can't name it, you can just listen in and see if it has any message for you. Let this sensation be in your body. When you get acquainted, you'll know what that part of you wants and why it's visiting, and you can proceed to soothing it. Reassure yourself and let the emotion pass through your body and imagine that it's going from you into the ground.

Pay attention to your posture and sit up straight. Imagine that there is a string of light going through your body from the top of your head to your pelvis. You will also need to focus on your breathing, and meditatively calm yourself, using your stomach to move the breath in and out of you. Relax your diaphragm as you inhale and suck in your breath by using your stomach muscles. As you do that, allow your emotion to safely pass through you. The more you do this, and the more you get to know your emotions, the more you can process them. This will graduate beyond those that are arising in the moment, but also those stored traumas that live inside your body.

Putting this mindful practice puts you into *adult mode*, where you can start promoting other emotions such as gratitude and compassion. This is not fake positivity, this is acknowledging and healing the difficult emotions and starting to promote a new mindset that will get you much further in life.

Chapter Seven: Craft Pain into Creativity

Everyday Life Creation

We tend to perceive daily chores as something that *needs to be done*. It's common to dread and procrastinate performing such tasks. But this significantly alters the experience, assigning negative associations with them. Instead, imagine fostering a different relationship with the mundane by practicing mindfulness. Start by focusing on the simplicity of it all, and the space it allows you to free up your mind. This offers an opportunity to listen to, and to calm, your thoughts and feelings. We might as well take advantage of it instead of doing things just out of necessity, especially since such tasks take up significant space in our lives. It takes practice, but try to be 100% present and to perceive the activity as a way to show love to yourself and to others.

The more you are able to sort through your thoughts and emotions, the more you'll start caring more about your surroundings, with an awareness of their psychological impact on your quality of life, and start taking pleasure and fulfillment from reorganizing, making space for what matters to you, and getting rid of things you no longer need or want. The more you practice this type of mindfulness, the more you'll realize how much better you'll feel when you've prioritised maintaining your priorities, and the reverence and sanctity of your sanctuary.

As I mentioned in Chapter five, I've personally struggled with this. As a child, everything was done for me. While at first I didn't consider it a priority, I have now come to see it as a gift to myself. I noticed the more of those gifts I gave myself elevated my energy levels and my capacity to give more of myself to others. I got there by learning how to be creative with my routines.

It's so true that our personal space is an outer reflection of what we're experiencing within. Now, imagine you are entering the home of someone you have just started to get to know. Their personal space is messy, chaotic, crowded with a lot of things they may need, and a lot that they don't need anymore. This can tell you a lot about them and their emotional state right away. Imagine their space was in such a poor state that it reflected they didn't have much respect for themselves to subject them to living in such conditions. And, someone who has little respect for themselves has little respect for others.

Imagine this person told you they were a workaholic. Therefore, perhaps they are too busy to prioritise organising and maintaining their living space. So, this could inform you that since they are not willing to make time for themselves, they likely wouldn't be willing to make time for you. Imagine being in a relationship with this person. If they didn't take the time to make a better first impression, it's likely they won't change, and this is what you can expect. If you don't want to spend time at their place, you'll spend more time at your place, where you can expect them to treat your personal space no differently than they would their own. So, you can also expect them not to change. If you try to improve their place, all the work will be on you. You won't find nourishment there.

If you are on a path to find a creative outlet through simplicity and organizing your personal space for the love of yourself and for others, it would be a compassionate kindness to yourself to find someone who shares those priorities. If you find that you know what you need in life, what is nourishing, and how aesthetics is important, but you struggle with knowing your "wants" and your purpose in life, you might need to work on speaking your truth and attending to all your emotions.

Now, on the opposite side of the spectrum, once your outer space is tended to, clean, and orderly, and you've created a peaceful space for yourself, it is time to look inward. Until you examine yourself more closely, you might not realize there are issues worth attending to. Let's call it your inner mundane tasks, and cleaning and organizing your inner spaces. If you find yourself frequently projecting outward, finding reasons to be resentful about the breaking up of a relationship or your ex, how does this projection mirror what is within you? Instead of hyper-focusing on that other person, hyper-focus on yourself.

Similar to your outer space, what is crowding your mind? Out of all of that clutter, what is it that you need and want, and what should you get rid of? Start by focusing on what you resented about the breakup and your ex. We often hyper-focus on the other person because looking in that mirror is more painful at times. Next, think about when you were in the relationship. Were you primarily serving your own interests? Or were you giving too much of yourself?

I find that these two problems are the main ones. This brings us back to one's inner and outer reflection, which more often than not can be traced back to their self-esteem. However, to find balance, try shifting your perspective. Rather than looking up to people or looking down at them, try to look at everyone at eye level and to see them as equals. This is a good practice towards embarking on a creative path towards embracing everything in your day-to-day life with mindfulness. The goal is to nourish your creative spirit and add a sense of fulfillment with everything you do.

The challenge is to not only address matters that are urgent or give you pleasure. You need to take care of those things you find yourself avoiding, omitting, that you find tedious, difficult, boring, and which through neglect often leads to bigger problems. You need to also find beauty in those things you often avoid. Otherwise, that ends up with another messy thing shoved aside, creating clutter in your inner spaces. Yet, when you declutter your life, approaching everything you do with as much love and positivity as you can gather, it opens your mind to the beauty of the simplicity of finding inner order and inner peace.

It's essential that we let our negative emotions pass through our bodies. And when they are passing through, it's important that we pay attention to the messages they are sending us, learn from them, and let them go so we can return to a homeostatic state of mind. Once you start adopting this mindset, creativity often follows and comes quite easily. Often, it takes the shape of an interpretation of our external world, and our emotional response, or inner reflection, of what we experienced in that world.

Professional Creative Expression

There are many people who truly believe they are not creatively inclined and don't have any artistic or musical talent. However, for most, this goes back to issues of self-esteem, self-image, and comparing their talent or creative expression to others. But, when you remove comparison and self-doubt, and find a safe space to express yourself, everyone is capable of creativity. Creativity often springs forth as an expression of your emotions. This can be through the work that you do, professionally or as a hobby. For example, someone who works with numbers and performs seemingly mundane tasks in their profession—if they enjoy doing the work—is capable of performing those tasks in novel and creative ways.

Of course, if you are currently working at a job that you don't find fulfilling, and don't have the option for creative expression, even through practicing mindfulness in your approach to the work, you're probably already feeling trapped and dream of working elsewhere. Similar to being in a toxic relationship, you need to look inward and start to declutter. What is preventing you from creating a lasting positive change in your life?

Yes, there are many circumstances which might prevent us from pursuing a career or position we truly desire. There is no shortage of terrible companies with poor practices and disturbed and demanding individuals in positions of leadership. But these are outward projections and are not an accurate reflection of who you are as a person. Giving up and surrendering to your situation is like staying in an abusive relationship and surrendering your power. Not to mention, being in a fear-based, anxiety-induced situation can paralyse you in a state of inaction. But if this is stifling your growth, and your creative spirit, for more than a third of your life, it carries with it the risk of leading to mental health issues.

It's important to prioritise creating room to express yourself creatively in every aspect of your life. One can start by examining what offers them fulfillment in their life, whether at home or at work or in their relationships. Perhaps you find fulfillment by helping your co-workers at your office job, whether through coaching or training, or just doing what you do for your job. This isn't people-pleasing, but simply genuinely giving when you can and caring. Or perhaps you innovate new approaches to how things are done at work, such as new systems and processes and strategies for streamlining and optimizing workflow.

All of it is creative because you consider how you feel at the workplace, how others feel, and what needs to be changed in order to have a better atmosphere. Making people feel things and striving for a better world is what defines art. The artist presents you with something that signifies what they feel to let you feel with them. But you can also take that piece of art and feel entirely different emotions sometimes. In this way, art is shared and owned by everyone that it touches. Perhaps Betty from accounting really liked your new filing system, was less stressed at work, and took that attitude with her to her family and shared it there.

When there is room for creative expression at work, it grants you the space to craft your emotions and energy into something tangible. And, by definition, that is art. And, innovation breeds more innovation, which creates a positive work environment, which attracts top talent. This is starkly different from working for a company that has a revolving door and a high employee turnover rate.

Crafting pain into creative art doesn't always need to mean painting or playing music. It's about bettering your life, and the lives of those around you, despite the pain. It is about creating purpose and value in our lives, despite the pain. By focusing on something meaningful, you are creating an avenue towards healing. Expressing ourselves creatively reflects self-worth, and forges paths forward that lead to rewarding experiences.

Relational Creative Expression

The power of creation is inside of us all. Everyone applies it differently, depending on their priorities, values, and perspectives. However, solely focusing on seeking fulfillment through a romantic relationship runs the risk of losing sight of other paths of fulfillment and self-reliance. This is especially dangerous when one shapes their definition of safety through the presence of a romantic partner. For example, a girlfriend of mine once shared that she didn't have a partner to pick her up from a hospital. In the absence of a significant other, she didn't want to turn to anyone else, or even fill out anyone as an emergency contact.

I then realised that it is quite common for people to believe that if they aren't in an intimate relationship with someone, then there is no one they can truly rely on. This is especially true of single women, who have it ingrained in them that if they have no partner, they have no protection. So what's left is the dysfunctional notion that they have to fend for themselves. To a degree, this is true. But when you look at your life and take account of all the people that matter to you, regardless of whether you are a man or a woman, there are always people on your shared life-path who are willing to help you, if they can.

Personally, my friends and family helped me more than any partner ever did. Perhaps this was because I didn't expect much from them in the first place, or didn't want to rely on them. But there is a need there to want to rely on a partner, and to depend on them. But what matters the most here is to accept that you can adapt, and will be okay, no matter what life throws your way. The universe doesn't give more than you can handle. I'm not necessarily preaching or practicing extreme self-reliance. It's important to ask for help. And if help is available, this creates the security and comfort to be willing to ask without expectations.

This is the path of creative relational expression. The more comfortable you feel with allowing yourself to rely on others, while accepting and feeling secure when help is unavailable, you can creatively build upon your relationships in unexpected ways. You can create a new sense of safety, security, and fulfillment, even with those relationships that aren't romantic by nature. This is true relational creativity. It creatively allows you the space for greater courage, feeling secure in your ability to express vulnerability, and learn more about yourself and how you navigate the world of your creation.

Experiential Expression

An extremely successful way of processing the emotions you are experiencing within is to simply give yourself permission to immerse yourself in them. If you are feeling sad or angry, give yourself permission to experience that, instead of carrying on and lying to yourself that you aren't feeling what you are feeling. Often, an excellent method for immersing yourself in those feelings is through experiential expression. For example, let's go back to listening mindfully to music.

Music is a great tool for processing your emotions. Music corresponds to our emotions, and it's okay to listen to some sad music from time to time. It not only validates what we feel but can also evoke those emotions so that we can let our body process them. If you are feeling anger, the principle is the same. Angry music is there for a reason because we all feel it at times. If you can play some instrument, that can also be an outlet. Try to match what you are feeling at the time through your music.

Whatever you choose to immerse yourself in, think of it as a cathartic experience. Go to a museum and see an art exhibit where the work reflects your inner state of being. If you are feeling lonely, go to a coffee shop or a library where you are unlikely to bump into anyone you know. Don't go there to be seen or to meet people but go there to be alone among other people who are also alone.

Artistic Creativity

If you enjoy expressing yourself through art, or are thinking about trying something new, I highly recommend it. This is another excellent cathartic approach for processing your emotions. When practicing art therapy, you don't necessarily need any *artistic talent*. All you need to focus on is expressing your emotions and thoughts.

Our brains are very effective at communicating complex emotions through symbols. We universally assign meaning to varying colors, patterns, and through the structure of what we are communicating through art. The same applies to music. These are inherent in our interpretation of the world and our experience through our bodies. Most music has treble and bass to it. The bass is the sound of our heartbeats within us. The treble is the sound of our nervous system, which we always hear, even in the utmost silence. The rhythm likewise can mirror our emotional state, and how our autonomic systems respond to what we are feeling. Slow and rhythmic tones—the relaxed state of our heart—can be relaxing or sad if they have deeper notes. And high-pitched quick tones and fast rhythms can be more exciting but also more anxiety-provoking.

I encourage you to communicate and express yourself from your adult self, in self-reflection and honesty, as opposed to your child-state which can lash out, withdraw, hide, people-please, or give up when not meeting an unrealistic standard of perfection. The act itself should be liberating, and it is extremely important to start creating without judging yourself, or what you are creating. The aim is to communicate and express. You need to acknowledge those emotions to be able to express them properly. Allow yourself to feel and experience what is going on within your body and mind as you remember those feelings and the memories tied to them.

The aim is not to show this to others, or seek approval, or fearing shame. You are learning, and what you accomplish through this form of expression needs to be approached with self-love, and love for what the work communicates. The second you allow what you've created to be misunderstood by others and what they project into their interpretation of who you are, you'll find your work will be judged, criticized, and run the risk of others suggesting how your work could be improved according to their vision or expression, and this defeats the entire purpose.

You are repairing your confidence and self-esteem. By seeking external validation for something you are working out with yourself will backfire. You are trying to understand and make sense of your inner cosmos. So you can't expect others to understand what you're still working out with your inner voices. Otherwise, you'll be creating more for other people and less for yourself.

The only reward you seek is what this accomplishes for you, and that is only discovered through committing to the exercise. You are expressing what is going on inside of you, so you are the only person who matters. Artistic expression can also serve as an amazing meditative practice. When exploring artistic expression as an outlet, the exercises and methods through which you choose to express yourself are limitless.

Here are some excellent art therapy exercises you can try if you're not sure where to start. You'll want to prepare by first creating a safe space for yourself before you start. I'd encourage you to have a nice and neat space. You can light a candle or incense and put on some relaxing music if you like. Your journey with art therapy is going to be very personal, so you need to feel comfortable and safe to allow yourself to experience your emotions.

EXERCISE 10
Art Therapy for Body Image

BODY OF POSITIVITY

Create an outline of your body (if you want to go big, make a real-size outline using your body on a bigger piece of paper!). Fill the inside with positive affirmations, images, and things that make you happy.

YOUR BODY-IMAGE

Draw what your body image means to you. I'm being vague for a reason. You want to give yourself a lot of space for creative interpretation.

Ask yourself, why is my body image important to me? What informs my ideal body image? When and where do I feel a boost in my self-esteem, and how does that reflect my idea of a positive body image?

'It can also be a drawing of you, whether informed by external factors or something completely different! It's up to you. By better understanding your concept of your body image, what informs that view, and why this concept influences your self-esteem, it will be easier to address those issues.

REFLECTION

If your body image is drawn from uncontrollable factors—such as others' opinions or comparing yourself to societal standards—it may be time to rebuild your self-esteem from internal factors rather than unrealistic external factors and societal expectations. Even if at one point you met that ideal, as you get older, it's not realistic to try to hold yourself to that standard. The aim is to view your body as a lovely vessel for your consciousness that grants you the opportunity to walk, hug loved ones, create connections, and live your life.

The aim is to shift your mindset to one where you offer *yourself* unconditional love, which includes self-love for your body, instead of comparing it to a product on the market. The moment you start comparing, you create a transactional atmosphere around your body. We are all susceptible to these trappings. Even if you try to live up to that unrealistic standard, and exercise on a regular basis and carefully monitor your diet, maintaining a balance between your mind, body, and spirit to meet that standard is not sustainable, nor motivation enough. Exercise from a place of mindful self-love, rather than a conditional transaction of meeting an expectation as a precondition for self-acceptance.

For example, I also always wanted a tattoo. Yet, I could never make up my mind on what tattoo would be worthy of getting. Yet, after I started dating someone who loved a particular style of artwork, it crystalized in my mind what the tattoo I wanted to get looked like. Yet, fortunately, before I committed to it, I realised the need I felt to alter my body came from a place of insecurity. When I started to work through it all, I realized that I truly didn't want to get a tattoo at all. Everything I thought I needed to communicate through a tattoo was already a part of me, and didn't need to be displayed for everyone to see.

Many people have different motivating factors for deciding to get a tattoo, many of which can be therapeutic. The point is looking at your own self-image, inwardly and outwardly, and finding love for yourself now, where you currently stand on your journey of living a creative life, and you'll continue to create and express who you are, where you are at on your journey, and where you want to go next. Once you figure this out and share it with the only person who matters—*YOU*—then you'll realise you're farther along your journey than you realised, and you'll meet people who are on that same road traveling next to you for a time, and in which case the only thing you need to share with them is that state of *being* on the journey.

EXERCISE 11
Art Therapy for Emotional Release

PART ONE: DRAW YOUR EMOTIONS

Before you begin to draw anything, sit down and close your eyes. Make sure to align your head, chest, stomach, and pelvis, and make sure that your arms and legs are uncrossed unless you choose a crossed-legged sitting position. If so, only your arms will be uncrossed. Now focus on your breathing and let your emotions come to you. Make sure that when you are breathing in, you push the air slightly down into your stomach so that you are not lifting your chest, and when you are breathing out, your stomach draws back in. Now let yourself experience whatever comes to you. It can be a memory, an image, or a sensation.

Next, ask yourself: "If this emotion could have a color and a structure, what would it look like?"

Once you've formed a rough picture in your mind, it's time to put it on paper. Aim to present your emotions through means that are presently available to you. Don't create reasons to put it off, like deciding at some indeterminate point to get the art supplies you'd need to accomplish this. Use whatever you have at your disposal. It's not supposed to be perfect; perfection is subjective anyway. This exercise is about transferring your emotions onto another medium.

Get to work. Once you feel like you have finished, meditate on how what you created makes you feel. Is it confronting, scary, or something else? Next, put it away and out of sight. Then meditate on how it feels, not having it near you. Some feel a sense of relief. If that's true for you, focus on the sensations of not experiencing that emotion you've found another home for through art.

Whatever medium you used to expel your emotions, if you want to permanently remove those emotions and what they are tied to from you, one option is burning them, whether it is art or journaling where you expelled all of your angry thoughts and negative emotions that were crowding your inner spaces. Anytime you need to declutter your inward spaces and want to get rid of the stuff you have no need for or don't want, consider using a safe-means for burning them. It is an exercise in letting go. In fact, the study found that when one group of people chose not to burn their emotional letters, they went on experiencing those difficult emotions, whereas the group that burned the letters improved their mental health. (Coslett 2024)

PART TWO: SENSORY RELEASE

You will need a big piece of paper for this part. Tape it to the table that you are sitting at. Sit up in your chair, and remember to align your head, chest, stomach, and pelvis in a straight line. And again, make sure that your legs and arms are uncrossed.

Start by acknowledging that your feet are on the floor and think about what it feels like to have ground underneath your feet. For the next five minutes, you are simply going to focus on your breathing. Breathe in using your diaphragm, expanding your stomach, and on the out-breath, you are softly drawing your stomach back in.

Keep your eyes closed and let your hand—or both hands—draw whatever feels right. Experience the sensation of holding your crayon or pen or pencil and moving it around. If it is a circle, half circle, a figure eight, or straight lines, practice whatever feels right to you. Be expressive. Imagine putting your emotion into the movement. Let yourself express whatever emotion comes your way with your movement while maintaining a straight posture as you perform this exercise.

Once it feels like you have finished, open your eyes. Do not judge what you've created, but simply spend time with it, listening to how it makes you feel to see these emotions outside of you, and what they mean to you.

Chapter Eight: Use Fluctuations in Attachment Style to Your Advantage

Every attachment style has its challenges and benefits. And, we all exhibit behaviors that can be either categorized as both an *avoidant* and a *preoccupied* attachment style. Our attachment styles change depending on the situation and the type of relationship we are in at the time. Both *preoccupied and avoidant* attachment style individuals typically internalise their partner's emotional state as their own, which can induce anxiety and a sense of uncertainty. When it comes to a person with an *avoidant* attachment style, those individuals will fear conflict, often people please and will have a hard time what they truly want and need from their relationships. Whereas more *preoccupied* attachment style people will know what they want but might use dysfunctional techniques such as blaming, clinginess or judgment to enforce their wants and needs to be met. There is also a *fearful* attachment style that tends to be a toxic combination of a *dismissive avoidant* and *preoccupied* attachment style.

There are differences in a breakup dynamic that can vary depending on which attachment style a person is in. So, in this chapter, I am going to share how to use your dynamic to your advantage and how to build up a more secure attachment style for your future relationships. We are going to explore how to use the benefits of your attachment style and how to work through the complex issues each attachment presents.

But first, let's briefly cover the different attachment styles, and at the end of the chapter, we'll cover what a *secure* attachment style looks like, and why it's worth aspiring for.

Anxiously Preoccupied Attachment

This attachment style is usually learned in a family where the parent or parents were present most of the time, but there were some inconsistencies with providing affection and attention, creating a dynamic where the child had to ask for it.

Someone with this attachment type is often preoccupied with their partner's emotional state, and how that impacts the state of their relationship. This often results in exhibiting excessive jealousy, neediness, and sometimes an increased demand for excessive amounts of attention. Nevertheless, those tendencies can vary from person to person. People with this attachment style are very in-tune with emotional cues and often invent new ways to attract needed attention.

Dismissive Avoidant Attachment

This attachment style is usually formed when a person is raised in a family where the parent or parents are absent, emotionally distant, or abusive.

Avoidants inhibit their emotions and needs. They often feel uncomfortable in intimate and vulnerable situations which require emotional connection, so typically withdraw from such intimacy. They have a more difficult time interpreting other people's emotional cues, as a result of them being disconnected from their own inhibited emotions and suppressed expression.

Fearful Attachment

This attachment style is typically learned from being raised in a pathological narcissistic family dynamic. People in this category often alternate between an anxiously *preoccupied attachment style* and a *dismissive avoidant attachment style*. The trauma they carry with them creates a need for instability. This typically leads to them creating a *pushing* and *pulling* dynamic from one relationship to the next.

Now that we've briefly covered the definitions of these attachment styles, let's analyze them all.

How to Heal When You Are the Avoidant Type

At the innocent beginning of my dating journey, like most teenage girls, I desperately wanted a boyfriend. Yet, when lacking any real relational experience or self-development, it's easy to end up with a broken heart or hurt feelings. So, it didn't take long for me to go from an emotionally available teen to being a dismissive avoidant.

Eventually, a guy that I somewhat liked took a fancy to me, and we started seeing each other often. We became very close. But now being an avoidant, I had no interest in commitment. Meanwhile, he repeatedly expressed his need for stability and became *preoccupied*. Granted, due to our lack of experience, we were both clueless about what stability truly meant. But that didn't matter. I was avoidant because of past heartbreak, and in the depth of my heart, I knew that he wasn't someone that I wanted to be with long-term. I wasn't severely avoidant. In fact, I was truthful about my lack of commitment.

Now, a severe avoidant would resort to people-pleasing in this scenario. Such a person would shut down and stop communicating altogether out of a paralysing fear of hurting the other person. Such a person would play-act as if everything was fine when it was not. But the dishonesty created breeds resentment and contempt within the avoidant, projecting their inaction and confused emotions on the other partner, blaming them for their situation.

As a young girl, I decided I was going to stay true to myself and simply didn't want to get too involved. I knew at some point I would leave that first relationship and was never committed to it or him. But it felt stable at the time, and being in any relationship felt better than not being in one at all. I offered myself a sense of stability I was looking for at the time and increased my sense of confidence. In a way, it was a survival mechanism.

Eventually, when I did indeed exit that relationship, I initially felt a great sense of relief—as is often the case with avoidants—that later took on the form of guilt. That person was never the right person for me, but I was too young to anticipate how this would all affect him, which later resulted in shame. Although there is nothing wrong with exiting a relationship that isn't right for you, it's not necessarily fair to the other person to remain in ambiguity with them. But once it's done, you need to come to terms with guilt and shame associated with it. And for avoidants, the most important part after a breakup is to recognize the pattern of avoiding intimacy and then trying to break free from it.

Befriending Your Emotions

When I first started in on my extensive meditations, I started feeling intuitive with my body in ways I didn't realise was possible. Emotions felt like impulses that dropped down from my brain throughout my nervous system. When I acknowledged them, they were quickly processed and washed over me. However, if I didn't listen, didn't interpret what they were communicating correctly, or was missing something, I could feel those energies cluster in my muscles, manifesting physically. Most people don't realise this until they practice being in-tune with their body in this way, but this is what is happening to all of us, every day, in our body.

So, anytime you find yourself slipping into a shame mindset, or going so far as viewing yourself as a bad person, this will detrimentally impact your life emotionally and physiologically, and end up thwarting your growth. So, let's get to know these emotions a little better—shame and guilt—and learn how to lean more towards guilt when making a mistake. The first step is to accept that these emotions will be there waiting for you, and it's best to not deny them. The more you ignore them, the more they will make their presence known. Rather, it's better to start to promote healthy patterns through inner dialogue with these emotions.

Befriending your guilt as a functional and useful emotion is the first step forward. When guilt makes its presence known, it is important to thank it. Remember, guilt is simply sharing feedback and informing you that you have room to improve and grow. The same goes for shame. Both of these emotions are simply letting you know that you *can* and *should* do better. So, rather than getting angry with those emotions or yourself, listen to them, thank them, and be mindful, gentle, and kind to yourself and those emotions.

What comes next is assuring them that you've listened to and heard the message they are sending you and have taken it to heart. Communicate that you realize you've made a mistake, and making a mistake doesn't make you a bad person. Once both guilt and shame are acknowledged and reassured, they will safely leave your body until they are needed again.

The Mirror of Truth

Relationships are mirrors. If you refuse to look into the reflection of the relationship provided, and refuse to learn from and acknowledge what it is revealing to you, you'll likely end up in a similar situation over and over again until you do. Avoidant wounds fester the more you suppress your feelings and thoughts. Recognizing what you are responsible for in the relationship, what you could have done differently, and where you withheld your truths are crucial to your growth. This is how we learn to not repeat the same patterns.

If you find yourself at first resenting, then later idealizing exes, and find yourself in the constant pursuit of *the perfect partner, you* might be trapped in an avoidant attachment style. Getting more comfortable with intimacy and with sharing yourself emotionally is the path towards healing and working on bettering yourself, and then refining, through your personal growth, what that *"perfect partner"* really looks like. Maybe, when you've done the work, and really hit your personal growth stride, you'll find what the *"perfect partner"* really looks like when you look in the mirror.

What it takes to get there is being on that journey with those who are at the same vibrational level. Because, no matter where you are in your growth journey, you are going to attract those who are at the same level of personal growth. And, if you haven't done the work, a *secure attachment* relationship will not be possible for you yet. As long as you are *stuck* in an *avoidant attachment style,* you will continue to hurt yourself and others. Perpetuating this cycle will continue to be a detriment to your mental health, and put you farther away from finding the fulfilling relationship you seek.

'Avoidants will only fully move on if they let go of their secretive expectations and their critical and judgmental world-view. And, if they are not ready, they'll often look for romantic partners who make them feel safe, such as those who are withdrawn or seemingly emotionally unavailable. Or, they'll find themselves attracted to those whom they recognize as being incompatible with, or whom they perceive as inferior in some way, which made them feel more secure and less attached. This allows them to keep the other person at an emotional distance.

Yet, this can often result in the other partner's confusion, leading to the other partner adopting an *anxiously preoccupied attachment style* who comes to crave transparency and understanding in the relationship. They'll end up asking questions, needing to know where they stand, frequently left with more questions than answers. This can evolve into being more clingy and exhibiting over-giving behaviors. And, when an avoidant labels their ex-partner as crazy and clingy, they are missing out on an important lesson. The more confused you are about your emotions, the more you will confuse others. Confusion breeds insecurity, and insecurity leads us to insecure actions and reactions. When your partner was preoccupied with the relationship, it's important to question whether you reinforced their behavior through your avoidance.

So, you need to be willing to constantly look at yourself in the mirror and openly and intimately share your emotions with the person looking back at you. Whereas, only looking at others' mistakes will only result in wallowing in your shame and finding blame in others for your actions. If you are still resenting your ex-partners and are not willing to change, you're not moving on. The only way forward is to change by forgiving yourself and others. This usually means leaning into your vulnerability. And not just in romantic relationships, but also in your friendships and familial relations.

Finding a compatible romantic partner is a physical, emotional, and spiritual need we all share. So often, this need comes with a fear of being alone. Instead of living in fear, you need to find the courage to be vulnerable and risk getting hurt. When you get hurt, you'll be okay. All you have to do is reassure yourself, be gentle with yourself, comfort yourself, and work through your emotions.

Once you feel you have made a little progress in this regard, don't stop. Making a little progress doesn't mean *you've done it* and can now move on. It's a constant practice. For avoidants, it's a constant practice to make a genuine connection, free of expectations of others, while giving your love freely and openly. Only after you can offer unconditional love for others will you start developing those deep connections.

Standards Versus Expectations

I often hear clients say, *"I have to have expectations, otherwise my partner will do whatever they want."* I usually respond to this with, *"You need to have standards and not expectations."* When you passively expect others to meet your expectations, you'll be disappointed, project that disappointment outward, will start to second-guess their actions, and stop communicating what you want.

Whereas having standards is more realistic. It accepts that not everyone will meet those standards, and you instead take ownership of your vulnerability by communicating your standards and being prepared for a potential rejection. This is an excellent example of forming a true connection, where you are not taking the other person for granted and give freely, expecting nothing in return. Try to think of expectations as a *rulebook* no one has read but you, that is specifically designed to protect yourself. When someone doesn't follow your *rules*, it gives you justification to be critical or to judge them. Whereas having a standard says *"What I need is X, Y, & Z. But, if you cannot meet that standard and cannot negotiate, I'll understand. It just means that we probably can't be in a relationship together, and that's totally okay."*

It's not always easy to adopt this kind of thinking. In fact, every bone in our body has a desire to secure in our relationships. Nevertheless, if you strive for it, you'll find yourself closer than ever to finding more fulfilling connections and will attract more secure partners. Once you let go of expectations and are willing to work with what is possible, you'll be able to make more grounded decisions. You'll also find yourself more accepting of others.

Allowing people to feel comfortable being themselves around you starts with being honest about who you are, who they are, about what you want in life, what you feel internally, and what you want from each other. Truth is both a privilege and a necessity in every relationship. You are not protecting yourself or anyone else by withholding it. Accepting even the most difficult truths can set you free.

Tightening Up Your Relationships

We can all heal to a certain degree without a relationship, but the truth is, romantic relationships typically offer emotionally charged opportunities you can't get elsewhere. However, if you think you are the severely avoidant type, you might need to start healing process by first developing close platonic friendships, while tightening up family relations. You can start by gradually talking to others about your emotions, such as people who are not extremely close to you. These can be friends who you don't have very strong ties with, work friends, acquaintances, or other social relations. Whereas starting with people whom you share a long history with—such as your parents—might be difficult to start with, the reason being that there may also be a great deal of suppressed emotions towards those people which you haven't yet resolved. Opening up to relatively new people often feels easier.

Sometimes parents force themselves into your situation, lack boundaries, and get over-involved. When this is the case and you feel overwhelmed, you need to raise that concern with them instead of avoiding them. You need to talk through those difficult feelings, especially when the connection is tightening. Also, if your parents are emotionally unavailable, simply recognize that for what it is, and create a safe space without expectations. Accepting their vulnerability is also important because if you don't do that, then again expectations will come back to bite you. Also, continue to assess your level of vulnerability. If you can safely say you feel comfortable talking about emotions with people in your life whom you are very close with, you are ready to restart your romantic search.

The Push and Pull Effect of Avoidance

Avoidants also have issues with feeling safe in conflict. They've habituated avoiding and people-pleasing, likely as a result of their parents not acknowledging their emotional needs. Once they feel like they're not being heard as a child, they might stop voicing their concerns, start keeping everything in, and end up developing poor communication skills.

Avoidants often develop *push-away* behaviors. They might start off by normalising such tendencies, justifying them as a need to take a little space. Other times, they may say something hurtful to push the other person away, and when confronted, claim they were *just joking*. However, what they often don't realize is that other people's bodies can physically feel that partner distancing themselves. Relying on these behaviors too heavily will result in others not knowing how to be around you, and many of those people will walk away, gladly giving you that distance and not coming back.

Therefore, eventually you'll need to develop some internal and external boundaries with people so that everyone knows how to be around you. The challenge is often to find a balance between setting those boundaries and expecting others to respect your space, while accepting that sometimes they won't realize that they have been stepping all over it.

In summary, avoidants need to lean into their relationships. They need to get comfortable talking about their emotions and learn how to have disagreements in a calm and collected way. They need to explore their own emotions, and how to feel comfortable being vulnerable enough to communicate those emotions to others. Letting go of expectations and developing calm standards will be crucial if you want to fully move on from your breakup and find a relationship that will be healthy and fulfilling in the future.

Avoidants often have depressive tendencies. Heightened awareness is often accompanied by anxiety. And when feeling anxious, especially about taking a risk of rendering ourselves vulnerable, we can often suppress those emotions as a defense mechanism. The problem is, when you suppress those emotions, they often transform into depression. And this simply turns one unconfronted emotion into another. So let those emotions out and lean into them. Befriend them. Listen to what they are communicating to you and be gentle and kind with those emotions. Assure and comfort them. Then start making changes where appropriate.

How to Heal When You Are the Preoccupied Type

While avoidants have a hard time getting their needs met through relationships, the anxiously preoccupied type throws their needs left, right, and center. On the one hand, this can be a positive thing, since you know how to be around them—that is, if they are not severely preoccupied and unreasonable about their needs. On the other hand, it can be hard to be assertive with someone who has a stronger and more demanding personality. When it comes to a person who has a more commanding personality, I like to refer to avoidants who have more commanding personalities as *emotional holders*. Whereas anxiously preoccupied types I refer to as *emotional over-expressers*.

By avoiding and not acknowledging the self, we end up suppressing the self and hold that negativity inward. In fact, holding emotions in can be harmful to the body, not just mentally but also physically, affecting certain muscle groups. Often hospital personnel can accurately predict who will end up with a positive cancer diagnosis based on how the patient carries their emotions in their body. Someone who expresses themselves less often ends up with a positive diagnosis.

On the other hand, *emotional over-expressers* tend to have a "strong personality" and end up smothering others by expressing their feelings through an emphatic vocabulary, wild gestures, speaking loudly, and using all sorts of methods to command attention. This is also unhealthy. What avoidant can learn from the preoccupied is to know thyself, and what the preoccupied can learn from the avoidant is to be more considerate of others.

What does being more considerate of others mean to the anxious-preoccupied type? It means not being needy, clingy, and demanding. It means not commanding others to validate you and make you feel more secure. That's why, if you are the anxious-preoccupied type, in order to heal properly, you will need to develop self-reliance, find multiple avenues to express your energy, and to learn how to generate your motivation from within. That is the work that lies ahead of the anxious-preoccupied type. To do this, you need to recognize the emotions that are driving this behavior. You need to start acknowledging how your preoccupied and insecure emotions are hijacking your actions.

As I said at the beginning of this chapter, we all exhibit behaviors that can be either categorized as both an *avoidant* and a *preoccupied* attachment style. Our attachment styles change depending on the situation and the type of relationship we are in at the time. So, it's common for someone who finds themselves shifting from an avoidant to a preoccupied to motivate themselves with how others perceive them. They may exercise more, work harder, and create more out of an insecure drive for validation, needing to show off, be praised, attract attention. A large percentage of this can even generate from a genuine desire to improve and be a better person. But as we discussed in previous chapters, seeking external validation can turn into a habit-forming fix.

So, you need to ask yourself, *"What happens to me when I can't get my needs met straight away?"* After asking yourself this question, pay attention to any uncomfortable sensations in your body. Listen to the parts of you that are *speaking* through those sensations. Ask how they are related to your self-worth.

Start questioning the images in your mind that you created which equate to your self-worth. Then ask what you've based those ideals on. We've all been there. During times of vulnerability, anytime I commanded and received external validation, it gave me a high. It gave me a feeling of matching that image I created of someone who was successful, attractive, driven, funny, worldly, and smart. Objectively, I was all of those things, but in reality, all of those things in some measure I created because of that little insecure girl that was bullied at school who still lived inside me. These things offered that little girl a feeling of protection. This is why it is important to not only learn to love others unconditionally, but to also love yourself unconditionally as well.

Emotional Self-Ownership

When you find yourself feeling difficult emotions towards someone, or are struggling to understand them or find compassion for them, it's important to recognize those are that mirror reflection on you again, and your unresolved problems. For example, anytime I find myself frustrated or repulsed by someone else's behaviors, I try to look at those individuals that are my *"no yet"*. What I mean by this is they are at a place in their lives I haven't yet been. I don't have a common reference point to relate to their experience and emotional state. So, since I cannot understand, I can't really judge them.

For example, I used to loathe clingy people. Inwardly, I labeled them as pathetic. That is until I became one. I loathed clinginess because there was a part of me that was clingy and needed to demand connection. So, anytime you find yourself judging someone, get interested in why. You might be judging something within yourself, driven by guilt or shame that you haven't accepted or befriended. There's a potential for growth here.

On the other hand, just as it is important to not judge someone who is beyond our referential comprehension, it's also important to not assume everyone thinks and acts like us. This falls under another common tendency of preoccupied types. They engage in presumptuous mind-reading and draw comparisons to themselves. Although we may know our own needs and wants intimately, we shouldn't assume other people are always similar. We shouldn't assume they have the same needs as us, or think like us. It's a normal human mechanism, but it needs to be replaced by a compassionate inquiry rather than constant assumptions.

People who are more preoccupied with relationships get their needs met by being demanding, expecting closeness, and being clingy. They also have difficulty waiting for their turn. When a preoccupied person exits a relationship, their immediate source of gratification is no longer there, and this can be traumatic for them. Therefore, a preoccupied type needs to find other sources of fulfillment without making them a permanent fix.

Healthy Outlets for Fulfillment

The main lesson for an anxious-preoccupied type to learn is to practice waiting their turn and to focus on meeting the needs of others at the same level as which they need their interests met. This requires reaching out to other people in your life while practicing a more reciprocal exchange with them. Also, when reaching out to friends and family, don't expect them to always be there. Remember, they are not there solely to meet your needs. So when they're not available, learn to accept it and find another surrogate relationship that feeds your needs.

There is nothing wrong with having needs. There's also nothing wrong with satisfying those needs. Be gentle with yourself and don't deny yourself what you need. Rather, be mindful and acknowledge what is driving those needs. Learn to accept that it's okay to not have those needs met at all times and there is no point to get upset at others when they're unable to meet them. Often, as soon as you let go, you'll serendipitously find that as soon as you give without expecting anything in return, your friends will start reciprocating more. This very thing happened to me and so many other people I know, and as soon as I let go, I met more people in a short period and I connected with them quickly.

This is why it's crucial to respect others' space and boundaries. When they tell you they are unavailable, learn how to take "no" for an answer. Push too hard, and you may end up rubbing them the wrong way, and then end up pushing them away. If you come on too strong, you need to be open to their feedback. In fact, you should welcome it. That feedback can help you grow, so be humble when feedback arrives. And, when you receive any feedback, don't respond straight away. Simply take in the feedback, carefully consider what it communicates to you and where it is coming from, and self-reflect. Only after you've taken the time to do that should you start considering how you want to thoughtfully respond. Being defensive will never help. You know your truth, and you need to learn how to communicate it gently.

The Therapeutic Impact of Empathy

Psychotherapy often focuses on the individual, but it's also important to take into consideration the context of humanity, and others' feelings and our impact on them. Through every experience and interaction, we affect each other every day, whether we like it or not. So when someone doesn't meet your expectations, it's important to react from a place of acceptance and compassion. This may prove especially challenging for some anxiously preoccupied types, and with practice, change comes gradually.

Closely examine your insecurities and your expectations, and try to change your perspective and relationship with those feelings. Instead of feeding those needy emotions through external validation, address them internally, without demanding validation from others. Start by coming to terms with the limitations of others. Instead, fulfill those needs with unconditional love for yourself, for those inner emotions and what the different parts of you are voicing, and handle this on your own. Then, when you are among others, don't anxiously wait for your turn. Be the person who listens instead of the person who is waiting to talk. Be there for others instead of expecting others to be there for you.

Learn how to self-soothe. Learn how to be okay on your own. This is crucial for learning how to be okay with not being in a relationship. Besides, for most anxiously preoccupied types, no friendship will replace the craving they feel for a romantic connection. But before you find that unconditional romantic connection, you need to make peace within yourself. Otherwise, those voices will not quiet down. You need to listen when your fear of loneliness comes around and says hello. You need to remind those fears that you need to do the work first. If you expect everyone to meet your needs all the time, that love will always be conditional.

You will need to have plenty of conversations with these feelings and inner voices. You are the only person who can reassure that part of you. To find that relationship you seek, you have to find a way to fulfill yourself. That being said, it is, of course, possible to heal within a relationship. But this will only be possible if you find someone who is as equally preoccupied with the relationship as you are. Yet, more common than not, an anxiously preoccupied type too often is more enticed and attracted to an avoidant. However, even though it's more challenging, it's often better to work on yourself individually, in order to achieve that state of feeling okay with being alone. You're trying to reach that state where you are confident that whatever happens to you, you'll be able to withstand it. That means reaching a state of becoming a Secure Attachment.

Secure Attachment

Someone with a secure attachment type was usually raised in a family that was consistently there for the child and installed this attachment style in them. This type typically feels comfortable with connection, intimacy, and vulnerability, especially when it comes to romantic relationships. Securely attached people have strong emotional regulation and communication skills, and they're typically not ruled by insecurity or fear of emotional closeness. They are better able to deal with rejections and breakups than people who have an anxious-preoccupied attachment style. They're better at recognizing their feelings and needs; therefore, they are better communicators than avoidants.

This is the goal of both anxious preoccupied types and avoidants and remains a possibility for everyone. Even if you didn't have that upbringing as a child, it's not too late for the adult in you to start giving the child in you what it needs. To get there, you need to work on softer communication, with yourself and with others, while decreasing insecure behaviors, and discovering where they are coming from, especially when it comes from your childhood experiences. The moment we forsake progress and repeat our mistakes, we start to get more and more anxious because our subconscious mind starts freaking out. Deep down, you know you set yourself back by repeating unhealthy patterns and by refusing to learn new things. That's an anxiety onset.

Anxiety Onset

It's important to not be ashamed of when anxiety and panic strikes. The goal is to move through it, learn from it, and try not to repeat it. In my life, I have experienced two strong onsets of anxiety. One revolved around academic achievement, and the inability to get what I wanted from it. I eventually found a way to work through this, but it took some time. The second instance, which I shared earlier on in this book, was related to not having the relationship that I wanted, and over-meditating as a fix. These occurrences heightened my awareness of my emotions as well as the emotions of others. This put me on the path to confront my emotions, to learn from them, and to becoming a better person.

As a person who has overcome severe anxiety, I can assure you that I am not unique, and you will overcome it as well. But to do so, you need to want to grow. And growth is what you need. What I learned from being an only child was, *"you won't always get what and who you want, make peace with it, and don't stop loving unconditionally."* Yet, even though you may not get what you want, I do believe we get exactly what we need in life. And, it's important to recognize when what we need comes along.

Often what we want at a certain time is not what we actually need, and that's why we won't get it. The moment you find your lesson, you'll learn from it and evolve. You need to make a difference for you, in whatever seemingly minuscule way that you can, in your life every day. There is no better cure than becoming a better human being. When that happens for you, things turn around... connections become more genuine, and you'll find more meaning in every mindful practice you perform in life, and unconditional love of self and others. Only then will your life be fulfilling. The rest is illusory smoke and mirrors. For this, you don't need to be happy 24/7; happiness is a poor purpose because it's fleeting. A purpose can also be a relationship where you give yourself unconditionally as well, and it doesn't need to mean that you do something super crucial for the whole world. For some, their purpose is simply being on that path to continually evolve and grow.

There's a serendipitous phenomenon that starts to happen when we are working with our emotions and striving to become a better person that captures the essence of personal development. This serendipity happens when we increase our vibrational level, and everything starts to align. All of a sudden, more and more "coincidences" arise, which help with processing the emotions that challenge us. You'll start bumping into the right people at the right time, and wonderful opportunities start presenting themselves left and right.

Chapter Nine: Address Your Generational Trauma

In this chapter, I am going to apply a model that aligns with my spiritual beliefs generated from personal experiences that seemed to transcend commonly accepted understandings of our world. As I share these with you, practice compassion with yourself, and practice opening your mind to whether this view and approach could work for you and be accepted by you. If you can't relate to it, then open your mind and explore ways in which you could apply and model this approach in a way that complements your own spiritual worldview.

Assigning Ownership to Trauma

As we move forward, the aim is to examine the emotions you are feeling, learn from them, and grow. But what happens when you can't unravel the complex emotions that your inner child is experiencing, and you start to open a dialogue with that part of you, and your inner child curls up into a ball, and chooses not to speak? Perhaps the fear and shyness of your inner child prevents them from communicating. What do you do when, for whatever reason, that approach isn't working? When this is the case, you will need to find another avenue for objectifying those amorphous emotions.

So who can you assign them to? Do those complex emotions that are creating turmoil within you even belong to you? How can you externalise those murky, indistinguishable emotions? How can you get them to offer clarity? How can you determine where those emotions come from? How do you empathize with them, honor and respect them, and then move on and grow, enabling you to break those unhealthy patterns?

Let's suppose they go farther back, to even before you were born. Let's suppose they are trauma carried to you from a past life, or carried to you by an ancestor. These aren't new concepts. In fact, reincarnation and ancestral trauma are concepts that go back millennia, and are still embraced across multiple cultures and religions around the globe, from Buddhism to ancient Egypt to modern spiritualism.

Admittedly, I understand how hard it is to accept, or even entertain, the possibility of such concepts if they don't fit into the spiritual model of your upbringing. Past lives were something I previously discounted and didn't take seriously. When people would say they had flashes or visions of something that happened in their past lives, I assumed it was just a dream or a byproduct of their imagination. Yet, it wasn't until my kundalini awakening delivered to me all sorts of experiences that I was suddenly able to accept varying concepts and beliefs, which I previously refuted.

So, having said that, the spiritual beliefs which I am about to share—in relation to the subject matter of this book and finding pathways to healing from trauma—may not necessarily align with yours. All I ask is for you to examine the value of what I have to share, how it pertains to healing and growing, with the aim of continuing down the path of becoming a more self-reliant, secure attachment type.

How My Experience Informed My Reality

Examine the value of what I volunteer here and ask how to apply these models to yourself. As I share how these principles fit into my spiritual beliefs, I ask you to bring with you an open mind, and to hear what I gained, and how you, too, can use similar experiences to your advantage. Remember, the aim is to heighten your spiritual approach to your life through an expansion of your understanding of the world, and an expansion of your personal beliefs, mythology, religion, doctrine, heritage, and lineage.

Now, let's go back to deciphering your trauma, and being able to personally address it. To do this, you need to atone with those emotions which are holding you back. Again, this is similar to doing your inner child's work. Yet, in this scenario, the trauma you carry with you might not even be your own.

The more I worked on myself, the more I was able to master my Kundalini energy. Now I'm able to move it around my body, balance my chakras, and experience a greater "high" from everyday life. With that also came abilities that I didn't know actually existed. This includes something I would have previously not taken seriously. I discovered how to release generational trauma. What this means is I am able to release trauma not only from my own life but also from past lives and previous generations of my ancestors.

Also, remember in chapter four, when I described a side effect of my Kundalini awakening? I mentioned that I had a heightened sense of other people's emotional states, and sometimes it was contagious, and easy to internalise and confuse as your own. The point is, there are many places where trauma that is not our own can find its way to us, and we mistakenly adopt that trauma and emotions as our own and end up carrying them with us.

When I started to learn about chakras when embarking on my Kundalini journey, I learned that a person's throat chakra is very much connected to speaking up and being authentic in the way you relate to others. When practicing Kundalini and moving through and aligning my chakras, I was surprised how massively affected my throat chakra was. Even more confusing was the fact that I never had issues with speaking my mind.

Now, I should mention that I am a Past Life Regressor Hypnotherapist, which means that I help people reach a hypnotic state where they can perceive their previous incarnations. Among those who believe in past-life-regression, there is the belief that the emotional and physical trauma you experience can be carried with you into your next lives, but it can also be carried through your family lineage from previous generations.

In a session I had with a fellow past life regressor hypnotherapist, it was revealed to me that in one of my past lives, my eyes, ears, and tongue were cut out. As grisly as this sounded, it offered me an object with which to process and break through that trauma. In many ways, in my present life, that trauma didn't belong to me, but I had inherited it, and now it was mine to deal with. Just as Alex, my Reiki practitioner, had trauma he was dealing with in his life, and those emotions were energetically bigger than him, to the point where they were contagious, and through osmosis, burdened me. Yet, similarly, his trauma didn't belong to me. However, that energy was now there for me to confront, to recognize as not my own, and then deal with and dispel it so I could unburden myself of it and move on.

Next, imagine that your great-great-grandmother had a broken hip that led to longstanding sexual issues, and now you have sexual issues which you cannot assign to any particular trauma or experience you've had in this lifetime. Most people have some sort of sexual generational trauma. In fact, I often meet with clients who have had a nice childhood and still exhibit sexual issues they struggle to deal with and cope with. All of these energies can be carried for generations, eventually finding a home in you, for you to deal with or pass down. Such problematic patterns and health concerns can remind us what needs to be addressed in order to become a better and healthier version of ourselves.

So, when performing your breathwork and inner child work isn't producing the results that you are looking for, consider reflecting back at past-life impressions, or talking to your ancestors and acknowledging their pain. This is called working through *transgenerational trauma*. To heal the generations of pain your body is carrying, you need to pay tribute to your ancestors and past incarnations. Try to gain an understanding of the trials that they went through. Integrate compassion into your approach. Allow yourself to feel their emotions, and then let them go. The idea is to rewrite their stories.

Examine the impact of how our ancestors and our past lives are shaping our reality, and not always for the better. Look at it as a test which those other incarnations kept taking and never passed. The universe gives us countless opportunities to retake that test. And once you pass the test, a new pattern will take form, solidify, and persist. This happens naturally once those difficult feelings are addressed, enabling you to move on from traumatic and unhealthy patterns. So, in this instance, you are retaking the test for them, and it's just a matter of transferring that pain.

The goal is to understand those traumas which don't belong to you, yet which you have been carrying. Treat that trauma with compassion, and then let it go. Again, you are decluttering, and releasing what you no longer need or want. Now, if you are not a believer in past lives or generational trauma and are struggling with this dynamic, open your mind to constructing a story that aligns with the trauma you have been carrying. Once you have a narrative that fits, then treat it with gentle kindness, and let it go.

Once you start to make real progress, it's similar to performing a deep cleaning in your home. The cleaner your home gets, the more you'll notice how dirty and cluttered it was, and how much more cleaning there is to do. The more trauma and unassignable pain you clear, the more you'll notice rising to the surface. So, when approaching this, it's a good idea to connect with your culture. Also, as you explore and learn more about your ancestral lines and connections, you'll want to pay attention to people who in some ways resemble you or exhibit similar patterns of behaviour. I call those people our "archetypes". When you recognize who your strongest archetype is, you need to examine what unhealthy patterns your archetype was cultivating, which you now seem to be preserving in your life. Then ask yourself what you could learn by changing those patterns.

You can also write a letter to your ancestors, acknowledging them and their emotions, while informing them that you are going to let go of them. Then, after you've written it, you can burn that letter later on.

EXERCISE 12
Visit Your Ancestors

Sit somewhere comfortable and close your eyes, focus on your breath, and sink into a meditative state. Now imagine you are walking towards your mom and dad—if you never met your family, that's okay. Instead, imagine their silhouettes. Stop in front of your parents, and imagine that all of your ancestors are standing behind them. Greet all of them with love and compassion.

Even if those family members or ancestors may have done you wrong, lovingly accept that this was the result of their own trauma and pain. You have chosen to take on the role of performing the internal work that needs to be done for yourself and all of your ancestors. So, treat each one of them with compassion, all the way back down the line. You are doing the work addressing the weight that has been passed all the way down the family line to you, choosing not to pass it further down the line. You are acknowledging what they went through without attaching yourself to their feelings. If you need to feel their pain, their sadness, shame, or whatever that ancestor is passing down to you, feel it briefly, without attachment, and quickly let it go.

You can also imagine that you are throwing that trauma into the fire, or packaging them up in a box of traumas. You can even say something of a symbolic nature, such as, *"Whatever from this box was mine and for me to deal with, I take on and decide to transmute into positivity. The rest I pass back to you with love and kindness."*

The possibilities are endless, and the story or narrative or experience you choose to live by is your own. The point is to identify the trauma, its source, or to assign a creative narrative, all the while determining why you are still carrying it. Once you are able to relate to the trauma, treat it with understanding and compassion, and gently let it go.

The Complicated Interplay Between My Now and Then

Often when we can't identify the trauma we are burdened with, we might not even recognize that we are carrying the trauma that is weighing us down. In such circumstances, we are feeling worn down and tired. When we find ourselves in a state of torment that mystifies us, we go looking for answers. And sometimes, those answers come to us in unexpected ways. For example, I once had something of a vision where I was addressing my ancestral trauma, making peace with my parents, and finding my current community. Many of the things in that vision later materialised and came true.

At that time, I saw a hypnotherapist who asked my subconscious a question, "When is Saskia going to meet her future partner?" The vision that followed in answer to her questions showed me a massive car park. Now, that isn't all that uncommon, and could be anywhere. So, at the time I didn't make too much of it.

However, my community gym is in the middle of a huge parking lot that overlooks another parking lot. Although that also might not seem remarkable, this ended up being how I met my Reiki Practitioner, Alex. So, I naturally wondered if he might be the future partner that the hypnotherapist asked about. Regardless, we were drawn to each other, and felt a real connection, being at similar vibrational levels. So, we worked together, and that's how he became my Reiki Practitioner.

Things started to happen to us at the same time. Health concerns and similar problems in life arose independently simultaneously. Then, when he started experiencing those deep and troubling family issues I mentioned in chapter four, I felt a great deal of compassion for him, which I confused for infatuation, and some of which I internalised and confused as my own trauma. Yet, at this time, I still felt a bit confused about that "future partner" vision, and entertained that perhaps Alex was that mysterious future partner. So, I asked Alex out on a date. But, I was a client, and he explained the conflict and declined my invitation. I'm happy he did, and we were both very mature about it and are still working together. And, in many ways, in the manner of which we are at a similar vibrational level and practicing Reiki together, one could define us as partners of a sort, just not as romantic partners.

As it turned out later, we came to realise we had a past life/ancestral connection, and that's another reason we were drawn to one another. What I also learned from my Kundalini awakening is when a person with strong Kundalini energy is in turmoil, we feel an exaggerated intensity of love and compassion for them. In fact, when in an awakening, everything seems stronger. Just like when someone was angry with Alex, I found myself annoyed with him, but couldn't say why. Later, we connected the dots. Eventually, we discovered our ancestral connection...

My Ancestor, who we'll name Cornelia, was sexually abused by her father. When she got pregnant by her lover, she planned to run away with him. But before she could, her father found out. Her lover didn't come to her rescue or to take her and her unborn child away with him. Instead, he abandoned her. Then her father poisoned her. After unknowingly taking the poison, Cornelia fell off the balcony. She died from a blow to the head, and her unborn child died with her, after surviving all of that sexual trauma.

Visions of these events haunted me, frequently leaving me to physically experience the echoes of her pain. In ways that are hard to describe, Cornelia greatly contributed to my personality, as did my grandmother. What my grandmother and Cornelia had in common was that they both gave themselves to men who failed to provide a sense of safety and security. This pattern persisted in the family. The women in my family entrusted their lives to partners who frequently didn't come through for them. So, Cornelia and my grandmother served as very strong archetypes for me.

When I eventually discovered Cornelia, and acknowledged her pain, as well as the pain of all the other women in my ancestry, I was able to replay the story of our ancestors, and change the narrative, relearning their lessons the right way. When you heal yourself, you heal generations backwards and forward. This is similar in concept to picking up on others' emotional or vibrational state. For example, at that time, my parents were struggling a bit in their relationship. But this too was generational. The women in my family were always very strong-headed, a bit volatile, and the men were avoidant.

During that time, when I was doing all of that kundalini work, my parents unexpectedly asked me to mediate for them. This was something they had never asked before. They had a strong enough relationship, yet still had issues. Part of which stemmed from my dad lagging with household chores and my mom being upset with him. Soon after doing that ancestral work, their relationship started to improve, and my dad started to be more emotional and less avoidant. This coincided with me feeling less insecure and putting aside my attention-seeking behaviours.

As it later turned out, my ex was also woven into this karmic story. In my relationship with him, it always felt like he was mothering me. When he was aiming to be nice and seemingly supportive and attentive, he was also withdrawing, pretending everything was fine, and looked at me as if the one who was creating problems for the both of us.

His past life trauma was directly correlated with Cornelia's mother. Cornelia's mother failed to protect her from her abusive father. Cornelia's mother also suffered abuse at the hands of her husband. Even though she tried to comfort her daughter, she often resented and blamed her, and remained voiceless. This led to her failing to aid Cornelia when she needed her most. Cornelia, and all the women in my family who submitted to unsafe men, were the foundation for my familial insecurities and similar inclinations. This doesn't mean the fault wasn't my own. On the contrary, I definitely promoted those patterns; however, I did so because those inclinations felt natural and familiar to me.

Finally, I was able to understand these repeating patterns in a new way and assign a source to them, which gave me what I needed to alter this pattern which has haunted the women in my family for generations. This was not an easy task. Many times I found myself just going through the motions, suffering fluctuations in libido, craving male attention… yet I resolved to break these unhealthy patterns until I could find a secure partner whom I deserve. And now, I finally understand what secure truly looks like. I learned how to feel secure in the way I interact with people, while always paying attention to the feelings and energies that are present in me at any given time. This is where removing ancestral influences led me.

Since then, I explored other past-life incarnations I've held, bringing to the surface multiple other traits I had issues with. The lessons I learned from those past incarnations aided me in addressing them, and transferring out that pain with the help of hypnosis and reiki.

When exploring your connections to your native culture and ancestral connections, it can help you understand aspects of your personality and sources of your behaviors which deserve closer examination. We are a result of our ancestors, and we are carrying with us the ancestral traumas we've inherited. It's also important to not expect change from your ancestors, including your parents. Expect nothing and receive everything. You cannot force anyone else to change. The decision to change has to be your own.

If you chose it, then you are the chosen one in your family line to instigate that change. So start thinking about it as rewriting their stories in this current lifetime. I know it sounds very fantastical, but every word is true. Be the black sheep of the family and choose a different direction, starting with working on yourself and breaking those patterns. Remember, the moment you increase your vibrational level, your external world will match it.

If you picked up this book and have gotten this far in reading it, you are most likely an open-minded and deeply spiritual person. However, if you don't consider yourself a spiritual person and this world-view is new to you, yet much of the other material in this book still speaks to you, that's okay. It's clear you have an open mind and are interested in exploring unique avenues to advance your healing and further yourself on your journey. So, consider what I offer in this chapter and invent unique ways to fit this approach into your life according to your own beliefs, upbringing, and doctrine.

Chapter Ten:
Signs that You Are Healing

We all want to believe we are doing better than we are. Sometimes even the smallest step in the right direction can feel like great strides. Yet, in all honesty, it's difficult to self-gauge what kind of progress we are making. I've come across plenty of cases where a client was adamant they've healed and moved on, yet it was apparent they were still suffering. I've been there, where I've told myself everything was fine, and ended up exploring new relationships too soon. However, when you backslide even just a little, feelings of shame and failure are common, which can lead to giving up altogether, or bouncing back into old familiar patterns.

If you are still holding on to the chance that your ex is going to walk through the door, and where you'd be willing to drop whatever you're doing just to be with them, there's still a lot of work to do. If you haven't yet moved on, you'll end up repeating the same patterns, and won't be able to make space for something new that better aligns with where you want to be.

Remember, your ideal partner is a reflection of your ideal self. And, until you raise your awareness, heal your wounds, release your trauma, and heighten your vibrational levels, any partner that comes along will only be drawn to those "lower vibrations". So, if you don't raise your vibrations, you'll end up attracting those same patterns that you are trying to move on from all over again.

To attract a better match or to make sure that going back to your ex doesn't end with a heartbreak yet again, you need to become someone who isn't reliant on a relationship. The moment you are truly okay with whatever the universe throws your way, you'll be free to enjoy your life. That's the paradox; you can't get what you want until you let it go. So, be honest with yourself. If you are still hung up, it's okay! Admitting it is important. It opens the door to healing whatever still needs to be healed within you, as opposed to wandering off to replay your patterns while generating more trauma.

I often find that people like to cheat in this department. I'm definitely guilty of this, and I see it in clients and friends all the time. We believe we are better off than we are because it is self-comforting to believe so. Therefore, we pretend, fooling ourselves while covering up the pain. This is not a solution, and it is not being honest or true to yourself. This will hold you back from the growth you seek, and you'll end up in the same situations over and over again. So, it is therefore crucial to make a practice of being honest and transparent with yourself.

EXERCISE 13
Honestly Better

Sit down somewhere quiet. Make sure to sit up and align your spine from the crown of your head down along your chest, stomach, and to your pelvis. You can choose a cross-legged position, or to sit down on a chair, or you can also lie down on a yoga mat. Have your legs and arms uncrossed. Focus on your breath, and make sure it's a calming breath, breathing into your stomach, using your diaphragm and not your chest. Continue focusing on that for a couple of minutes, studying the emotions and thoughts that arise. Allow them in and get curious about them. Once you are sufficiently tapped into your subconscious and attuned to your impulse emotions, start asking yourself questions listed below.

1) Do I feel like I need this particular relationship to feel complete and fulfilled?
2) Would I compromise my boundaries for this relationship again?
3) Would I still consider this partner in the future if I was already creating something meaningful with someone new and potentially better for my personal growth?

4) Do I feel like I can handle any potential scenario that life throws my way and that I'll be able to bounce back to a good state in any case?

These answers are not absolute indicators of your healing, but they will give you a good idea of where you are at with your healing journey.

This is also where seeking feedback can be incredibly useful. Find someone who is different from you, who you trust and find credible, who has a different world view, and ask them how they think you're doing. If you are a timid and people-pleasing type, ask a friend who is more outgoing, confident, and maybe even a bit more selfish than you are. A person who is the polar opposite of you and has a healthy personality will better see you from a perspective that you perhaps can't see yourself.

However, such a person may not always be available in our lives. In which case, you'll need to monitor yourself more closely and carefully study, document, and assess your behavioral changes after the breakup. This is why journaling can come in handy, where you can look back at your journal entries and compare how you were doing to how you are now. Another method for self-gauging with a level of accuracy and a heightened level of self-awareness is trying to create an image of yourself when you are at your absolute best. Where you're thriving and in the best mental health, feeling grounded and secure. This is your reference point. Another reference point is to imagine the future *you*. This is who you want to be at the end of the path you are on to becoming that person.

EXERCISE 14
You Upgraded

PART ONE:

You will need a pen and paper for this. First, write down what you value in life and rate each area from 1 to 10, where 1 is *not significant* and 10 is *the most significant*.

Here are some common life areas that you might value in life:
- Spirituality
- Money and Finances
- Career and Work
- Personal Growth and Learning
- Partner and Love
- Family and Friends
- Community
- Environment
- Fun and Recreation
- Health and Fitness
- Politics and World Situation

Rate each of them from 1 to 10. See which numbers are the highest and write down how you plan to improve them. Think about your life's purpose. When do you feel the most fulfilled? Where do you see yourself in 5 years? Write all of this down and describe this person. What do this person's habits, living situation, friend's group, and work look like? What is it like to be this person? Now write down the steps you can take from here to become this future *you*? You want to be as specific as possible.

PART TWO:

Now that you have a baseline in mind and you have a plan for manifesting the future version of you, you are ready for this difficult assessment. You will need to compare:
- The future *You*
- The *best version of you so far*
- Who you are currently?

Next, draw a scale line. The far left side of the line is you at your lowest point. At the other end of the bar is the best version of you so far. Then, place a mark of where on that line you honestly feel like you are between you at your lowest and you at your best so far. Lastly, outside of that line, place a mark farther up that indicates where the best version of the future you could be in the future. And then count how many of your scale bars it would take to get there. This is similar to a scale bar on a map which is meant to help you measure the distance between two points.

PART THREE:

Next, you are going to shorten the distance between those points—where you are, the best version of you so far, and the future of you. To do this, think about those behaviors that are definitely not going to take you to your best-self. Then you need to establish what in your routine is to be discarded and what should be added in order to be on the path to the baseline and ultimately to the future self. Be as specific and as detailed as possible when it comes to this analysis. Every small behavior matters. As soon as you think of those habits or routines, you need to clear out, you'll determine how much distance those take up on your scale line to getting to where you want to be.

Start with any atypical bad habits, such as sex, alcohol, drugs, unhealthy dating patters, or any other escapes or fixes you are relying on. Even seemingly *neutral* or *healthier* habits, such as social media or being seen at the gym, or other forms of exhibitionism. Even if you go to a bar with your friends, and you aren't *drinking that much*. It counts if you are going there to look your best and hope to be noticed and seen to feed your ego.

I'm just as guilty of this as anyone. It's perfectly human to fuel that need. Yet, an interesting thing happened. As soon as I entered a relationship that felt like a step in the right direction, I was suddenly more aware of those tendencies and stopped them. For instance, I wasn't initially aware of my impatience when I was engaged in conversations with my friends. I was always waiting to talk instead of truly listening.

As soon as I found myself in a secure relationship, I no longer resorted to my fixing behaviors, such as driving recklessly, posting on social media, or hanging out with the wrong crowd. I even found drinking less appealing. In some ways, that relationship healed my insecurities, and in other ways, it masked them. However, as soon as that relationship ended, I wanted to fall back on those old and tired fixes and patterns, seeking comfort in those things which I once thought made me feel good. The thing is when you truly recognize you are using a certain behavior as a Band-Aid to cover up old wounds and trauma, that Band-Aid just doesn't stick anymore, and keeps falling off. And the wound is still there.

Although that breakup was painful, it allowed me to heal to the point that those old fixes weren't enough. So, I forced myself to develop healthy behaviors instead of relying on fixes. After that, each time I left a relationship, I continued to choose healthier patterns, enabling me to be a more compassionate and loving person. Finding beauty in hardship is rarely easy. But it does offer you a chance to make your world, and the way you look at it, more beautiful.

Heartache and personal turmoil simply make what you have to work on more apparent. If your reflex is to deny that anything is wrong when relating to yourself and others, you need to be more honest with yourself and go back to Exercise 13. Everyone has room to grow, without exception. If you are stuck in a loop, experiencing the same type of breakup with the same type of people over and over again, it's a clear sign that you are stuck. If after each relationship you find yourself blaming them, glossing over your feelings, or wallowing in them, you might be struggling with mustering up the courage to process them and embark on your healing journey. That means you are bottled up, and perhaps fearful of feeling the pain you are carrying. If that's the case, it might be time to break the dam and release the flood.

Breaking the Dam Releases the Flood

When I was going through my tough Kundalini awakening, I started to become more in-tune with my body. I came to understand how emotions got stored in my facia (connective tissue between the muscles). How treating someone with true love and compassion physically affected me.

How, when I got upset at something, not only I was upset at the moment but I could feel other *energetic remnants* of that emotion in my body long after, literally shaking and trembling throughout. This is called an *emotional flooding*, and is something all of us experience from time to time. Relationships are especially prone to these.

Initially, at the end of that relationship, I didn't recognize myself. I got flooded very easily and felt like I wasn't in full control. When you are working against your emotions, fighting them, you'll be fighting against the flood. But there will continue to be cracks in the dam. However, once you swim through the flood of those emotions, start working with them, allowing yourself to feel and process, you will not be flooded as easily. The goal is to still those waters so that you can see yourself clearly through them.

If you don't experience emotional flooding, it might just mean you've built a pretty good dam, or have buried that trauma so deep inside your body, it's just waiting to be shaken up again by someone new. It might come out by overreacting when you feel hurt or offended, or losing control of your temper and your emotional responses. Then, when you calm down, you feel shame for your volatile responses, which fuels those self-afflicting emotions. If you want to break free from this pattern, which feels like an endless spiral, at some point in your life you will need to break it all open to free yourself to having a better life. It really doesn't get better if you keep locking your feelings away. Because if you remember well, we attract people with a similar level of trauma.

If you are hiding from your emotions and feelings, denying your opportunity to grow and move forward, refusing to break free from being stuck, and not living your life in a way that keeps you on the path to being *you at your best*. If you are stuck but are no longer affected by emotional flooding, you are "dead inside" and yet hyperactive on the outside. This is a fast track to bitterness, distrust, and toxic relationships. It leads to anxiety, depression, mood swings, and communication issues.

It's natural, throughout our lives, to feel overcome by difficult feelings that keep us from living the life that we want. We all end up repeating the same patterns and falling into the same thought spirals that hold us back from growth and change. However, through practice, we can all use certain vibrations which have the opposite effect and promote healing.

As I started to peel back the layers, improving my communication skills with myself and those around me, my body started to feel healthier, energized, and my senses enhanced. I made the choice to heal any resentment I felt towards my ex-partners, my parents, my friends, and anyone who has ever "wronged" me. The more I understood the underlying issues and difficult feelings behind those resentments, the easier it was to let go of them. I chose forgiveness as a path to moving on, and I chose to release my romantic pain as well as all the rest.

Again, you have to self-gauge against your *future self*. And when envisioning your future self, it is important to visualize an ideal that they may not be wholly ideal. This means far more responsibilities and healthier habits that your *future self* has to maintain and uphold. And sure, they'll be having an easier time of it than you are, but the things that are keeping you from that healthier path aren't a problem for them.

I truly believe that the ending of a relationship is a unique opportunity to heal more than the wounds from that relationship, but to clearly examine what older and more buried issues that rose to the surface as a result of that relationship. So often, the power of romantic relationships can correlate with parent dynamics, sibling dynamics, and your relationship with yourself, and all the problems with all of your relationships, but in the most intimate and vulnerable ways. In this regard, no other type of human relation is so powerful as romantic love and covers all facets of life such as the sexual and intimate. Every breakup can yield clues to unlocking your potential and purpose.

As soon as you start healing, you'll recognise it was never really about your partner. It was always about you and how you related to the world around you. It was about your relationship with your parents or your upbringing. Even those influential parental figures were loving and nurturing. It's about access, nurturing, safety, protection, and whether crucial developmental needs were met. It was about your expectations, your fears, vulnerability, and trust. How these impacted the shaping of our world and character can influence nearly every decision you make with all of your relationships throughout your life.

The best measure of your healing is to see what kind of people you are attracting, and not solely in a romantic sense. This applies to even casual interactions. If healthy and balanced people gravitate towards you and enjoy your company, you are definitely on the money. But if you see that strange and unhinged types are resonating with you, and you with them, this is an indication that you still have plenty of work to do before manifesting a healthy and stable relationship.

Spiritual Signs of Healing

I personally believe we are in the midst of a tremendous spiritual awakening on our planet. For the first time in history, we have ample time and resources to work on ourselves; personal development, becoming better people, and developing more compassion for ourselves and others. These pursuits raise our vibrational levels. According to quantum physics, everything is vibrations, including our bodies. An atom's structure, from its nucleus heart, to its electrons and protons, and sub-atomically quarks, all the way down to string theory—every foundation of matter—is in perpetual motion and vibrating. Entire buildings can be destroyed with a properly matched vibration. Even useful and practical technological devices can be harmful thanks to the frequencies they emit.

Yet, when you're stuck in those bad patterns, and everything is dammed up and locked away, and only coming out in negative outbursts followed by guilt and shame, your body can still physically feel those lower vibrations as well, which can be self-destructive. We too vibrate at a certain level, and the more emotions we pent up inside, the more health concerns we will encounter, and the less space we have for compassion and happiness. Remember in Chapter 8 when I mentioned how hospital personnel can often accurately predict who will end up with a positive cancer diagnosis based on how the patient carries their emotions in their body?

Pain is interlinked with pleasure. If you are unwilling to move through pain, you'll find no pleasure, and be stuck inside the pain you're bottling up inside. And more pain will come. That's why there is so much pain in our society. People are either unwilling to face their problems even when they have time and opportunity to do so, or they're expected to keep their pain to themselves, to bottle it up, and to carry on, as if that is the only show of strength. Yet, it is only when you have the courage to be different and face that pain and move through the flood that the freedom, rewards, and love will flow your way.

Our body is capable of healing itself, but only once the stress and trauma leave the body. On a biological level, it's been proven how stress affects the body. When we release stress, there is space for our natural DMT to be produced. The body wants to heal itself, to process those feelings, and to raise your vibrations in a positive way. This only happens if you allow the release to happen, and that includes going through the pain of experiencing those feelings and reliving traumas in a safe and controlled environment. And, a break-up is a perfect time for this because it gives you clarity on what you need to focus on and how to approach your healing journey.

And remember, your healing journey isn't just about your emotions, your relationships, your past lives, or the generational trauma passed down to you from people you've never even met. It's about your body, the energy you are carrying with you, and your future self, and how their fate is in your hands. It is about forgiveness, decluttering your emotional load, and letting go and releasing feelings of judgment, resentment, heartbreak, insecurity, betrayal, and being willing to walk through the fire. As soon as you let all of those burdens burn away, what is left is a better version of you.

While undertaking this *trial by fire*, you might find that old patterns and bad habits are no longer as appealing, leaning towards healthier pursuits and more authentic connections. You'll form new friendships, and new opportunities and people will come your way. This is because you are attracting things and individuals at your new vibrational level. You have *created space for the new*.

There is so much more love to be experienced in life, in this world, once we dare to walk through that fire. Keeping the flood at bay will prevent you from experiencing habitual unconditional love. Once you survive the flood and walk through the fire, your world view is shifted to that of a survivor of the flood and the fire. Your world is made anew. Serendipitous events, new people who are also survivors, and fresh opportunities are a true sign that you are healing, that you've unstuck yourself. This comes with a disinterest in those same old patterns, feelings of happiness, and feeling more fulfilled.

This is the first step towards the future you, who vibrates at a level that will attract the future partner you dream of. This person doesn't complete you. They resonate and vibrate at the same level as you, and understand you in a different way than you've experienced before. Relationships where both people work on themselves are healthier and long-lasting. When two people are on paths to mutual self-growth, they don't typically become stagnant. Someone who is on a journey towards becoming an improved version of themselves will be able to share insights from their journey with their journey-partner, which they'll both appreciate.

Now that you have an understanding of how far along you are on your journey, you can turn the page and explore whether you're ready for your new romantic venture. Otherwise, stop here and continue releasing those pent-up emotions. Remember, it is okay to not be ready yet. If you go into dating too quickly, you run the risk of pushing that trauma back into your body and covering it up with band-aids, instead of using this opportunity to go deeper into your pain, to more closely examine those wounds, to apply the only medicine that can treat it, which is awareness and self-love.

Nevertheless, perhaps you haven't been hurt enough! If you need to go back into those situations and people open yourself up fully and experience the full gravity of it. At some point you will hit the rock bottom and from there you can only go up. That's what I have done and that led me to my awakening. Studies have shown that people who are wholehearted in that way have a better mental health and resilience. Dare to be hurt massively and pick yourself up, this versions of you will be able to take anything and anyone on. It will also be able to find a healthy, connected and fulfilling relationship.

Chapter Eleven: Signs that You Are Ready to Get Back Out There

Cutting The Cord

Let's remember that there is no such thing as a 100% healed individual. It's constant work, which you need to vigilantly continue for the rest of your life. Yet, if you find yourself doubting your readiness, examine whether you have truly cut all possible cords with your ex-partners. Even the most seemingly insignificant things can have an emotional transference attached to them. For example, keeping ties with your ex's friends on social media. You might justify this with, *"I can be the bigger person,"* or *"They're nice people. It doesn't feel right to block them."* Anytime you post on social media, do you secretly hope your ex's social circle might see how well you are doing without them? Is this a fix, or is it a means for seeking validation? If this is true, you're not really keeping in touch with them, and it might be best to cut those ties and move on.

It's okay to prioritise yourself, and protect yourself from unhelpful patterns and detrimental thoughts and behaviors. It's okay to cut ties with people, things, and situations if they are not serving you in any meaningful way. Stop thinking about what other people think and want from you. Sometimes that's just an excuse anyway and how you might end up propagating the same bad habits in your life. Rather, be honest with yourself and cut the cords to any attachments or feelings that are holding you back. Stop looking for external validation. Once you feel it on the inside, you'll instinctually believe it and have no need for external confirmation.

Hermitage and Stillness

We all need periods of stillness and hermitage. I myself went through a period of reflection for about 7 months before making myself romantically available again. Yet, if you lock yourself up at home and simply hang around waiting until you are *truly ready* for someone new, you might as well buy a few cats and throw away that key. But building resilience is much more effective than trying to regain some sort of elusive hope. Waiting around for something to happen blocks important lessons and emotions from coming through, and thwarting you from healing further and reaching the next level of awareness. That's when you need to examine whether you are isolating as a course of self-reflection, or if you are hiding and protecting yourself from the outside world, trying to keep anything from coming in.

Sometimes we are in so much pain that it's hard to trust the world again. As I mentioned, we are never 100% ready for everything that comes our way. It's definitely important to take time to work on yourself, to find stillness and self-reflect. But it's also important to re-engage in action, in adversity, and to allow yourself to experience all the excitement that life brings. We can't wait out the pain while in hiding. Hiding from the experiences that remind you of that pain only keeps you from facing new trails, which, like everything else in the world, simply comes with the risk of getting hurt. Working through your pain diligently after a break-up requires continually acknowledging any feelings that arise and allowing them to pass through you, as you practice connection on every level available to you right now.

So, if you truly found that stillness and your recuperation gave you a new insight and renewed strength, why wouldn't you put it to the test? Finding trust in the world again only comes about when you trust you'll be okay at the end of each situation you face. You need to form a real and long-lasting trust with yourself. Yet, if you refuse to put it to the test, you are attaching yourself to a limited convention, and the universe will eventually put you to the test anyway, whether you like it or not.

You must be ready to accept the risks involved only after you open your mind and heart and truly trust yourself. That's the only way to train your intuition. If you look back at your ex as instrumental in having helped you adjust your course and move away from what you don't want in a partner, try looking at it a different way. Maybe the credit wasn't theirs, but yours. You embarked on a new type of relationship. And, the situation that unfolded from experiencing a relationship with that type of person opened your mind to what is possible, and what type of relationships are available to you at each stage of growth. Those were your choices, and you deserve the credit for having risked getting hurt, and having gained new insights from that experience. This view suggests you have that and more to look forward to with your next relationships.

Having learned those lessons, you'll be better at recognizing who is good for you, and won't settle for someone who resembles your ex or the previous trauma-patterns you've broken away from. You'll be looking for an upgrade, and will only find it when you've upgraded yourself. Not to mention, thinking that the world will at some point stop throwing curve balls your way is yet another naïve fantasy.

The Commercialization of Romantic Ideals

The idea of romantic love in Western cultures has evolved and been glorified throughout the centuries. We put so much emphasis on finding *the one*—that perfect partner whom we'd abandon everything for, even our own individuality. The idea of *the one* is problematic. We tend to believe what we want to believe when it comes to this label, instead of seeing that person for who they are. They are our projection of an unrealistic ideal. I often see people giving this tag to a person that is not suitable for them, and then that label is even more difficult to remove.

Perfection is subjective and we tend to compare ourselves to others to seek it. We can still work on ourselves and develop while in a relationship. It isn't necessary to wait for a relationship to come along that is the spitting image of perfection. However, if you're clinging onto the idea that love is a fairytale, where you will be rescued or swept up off of your feet, you might still be stuck in your trauma loop. To find out, simply ask yourself the following question: Do you need rescuing? If so, why can't you rescue yourself?

TV often feeds us this image of idyllic perfection that is bestowed upon life when you find *the one*. The idea that someone else completes you suggests that you are incomplete, imperfect, not whole, which conveys being inadequate, needy, and incapable on your own. The only person who can complete your journey is you. The only person who can decide who you've been, who you are, and who you choose to be is *you*. That is *not* up to someone else to do for you, or to decide for you.

The first step of being ready for a new romantic adventure is to understand that relationships are not there to save you from anything. They are not there to just make you feel warm and fuzzy. Just because one particular person loves you might not be enough to spark and keep your self-love lit. You need to be responsible for your own growth and self-worth. Of course, connections with others can enhance this, but only if your "self-worth generator" is already on.

Some time ago, I came around to revise and update my online dating profile. Just as I did so, I started ruminating about my ex. After that, I decided it would probably be better if I were to meet someone organically, and shifted my attitude to thinking, "the right person will come into my life at the right time while I continue to do my thing." Admittedly, I'm still uncovering new lessons which I still have yet to learn, but they are getting less and less frequent, and more connected to broader ideas. For example, there are greater lessons to learn, such as relationship choices, especially when it comes to male and female relations. Such as being more discerning and aware of a woman's safety as a priority in a world where men usually have a physical upper hand and cannot always be trusted. Nevertheless, I believe that now I have fully moved on and if I was to give a rough timeline for healing it would be about a year from the break up. I can truly say I have finished my healing journey at about the same time when I should have left that relationship the year before. But more emotional space and a new direction came about a year from the break up. I believe that healing has an ending but needs to be maintained. I can physically feel lighter, my body emptied out of stagnant energy, I became very flexible, unaffected by foods that use to give me issues, my flat foot, scoliosis and immune issues disappeared and never came back. My body looks better than ever before and it's easy to maintain it. I'm planning to keep up the work I'm doing but I can finally say that trauma has left my body and I just need to flush out daily issues.

The realization that I don't need a relationship to be happy and fulfilled was one of the greatest things that ever happened to me. I was putting too much emphasis on romance and not enough on friendships, which didn't seem as fulfilling at the time, only because I hadn't explored myself deeply enough. In order to feel closer to others, you first need to start with nurturing your relationship with yourself. We are only able to be as close with others as we are with our complete self. I believe this is one of the greatest issues within the current dating scene. Where the work you've done on yourself is incomplete, and you expect that other person to complete you.

Twin Flames Versus Karmic Connections

In spirituality, there is the idea of a "twin flame". It's explained as one soul divided into two people who are perfect mirrors of one another. Some people consider this the ultimate love. Nevertheless, an intense and fiery romantic connection is one that enables you to remain stuck in old patterns. The ideal of an ultimate twin flame is intense and is supposed to feel right and push you to become a better person. If this isn't the case, it's just fiery and intense, which runs the risk of becoming increasingly toxic, exhausting, and doesn't really align with your twin flame ideal. Those relationships are usually very fiery and passionate but blow up quickly, only increasing your awareness of self and what personal healing you need to prioritise.

After a relationship that ended which I initially labeled as my *twin flame*, I imagined us getting back together eventually, once we're ready and we've dedicated some time to our individual personal growth. I wasn't interested in a simple soulmate relationship. Later I realised I was locking myself into a fairytale *twin flame* ideal, which was holding me back on my healing journey. Giving that person a label of *one and only* was a big hurdle that I had to overcome, having placed too much faith in those *signs* that he was the *one and only*.

We were really good mirrors for each other. Quite often, the person you are with will mirror all your problems, and that can be overwhelming. But mirroring problems doesn't always indicate growth. And this can lead to confusion. This isn't dissimilar to a trauma bond.

Similarly, often people run away from deathful relationships because they are afraid of all the things that they saw in the mirror that need to be addressed. This is why self-awareness is crucial. If you are not being consistent with self-awareness, health routines, and compassion towards yourself and others, you will encounter increasingly difficult situations and emotions that will shock you to your core.

There's also an important distinction between a *twin flame* and a *karmic connection*. For example, once I embraced the path of bettering myself, new and interesting people came into my life. A lot of men that I previously didn't believe existed. Men who were generous, funny, attractive, health-orientated, spiritual, successful, contentious, and courageous. They've become my friends, and I feel comfortable in their presence. They've helped me realize that there is no *one and only*.

Prioritising yourself and your emotional well-being will invite the right people to you.

Once you break free from unhealthy patterns, start to create peace within, and walk slowly but surely towards health, self-love, and fulfillment, you will no longer be bound by an obsessive need to be with someone. It's perfectly fine to wonder what your next romantic adventure will look like? In fact, I encourage you to continue to live with that question. Continue to get excited about it, especially as you come to realize more and more what is possible with each stage of healing and growth you experience. Get even more excited about it as you increase your capacity for self-love and self-acceptance.

There are many people that will come along and seem like a match for what you want. Yet, those individuals might not be vibrating at the same level as you. This is why it is important to continue working on and prioritising yourself. When you undergo massive changes and continue to work on yourself, your ultimate tribe of people walking along that same road will form. Your journeys will overlap and you'll all be walking side by side. In fact, similar to that partner who situationally revealed to you what was possible, so are your fellow travelers. Yet, these journey-partners don't need to be romantic partners. Friendships can be just as insightful if we let them.

Spiritual Activation

My spiritual activation was sparked into motion through love and a search for romantic love. But yours might be something else. Always the source of one's spiritual activation are the lessons they are being forced to learn, or re-learn. Once you look back at your lessons—whether it is some sort of attachment, your health, your outlook, your children or parents—breaking away from your old unhelpful patterns and starts suddenly seeming so much easier than you previously thought.

We don't always choose our paths. Often, they seem predetermined. Looking back at my previous romantic ventures, I can trace back each great improvement, like stepping stones leading to where I am and continuing on from where I stand. That's why I stopped looking at relationships as a cure. Now I'm looking for someone who will keep me company on my journey of self-development. In fact, I would like to refrain from saying that I'm *looking*. Let's rephrase that to, *I'm willing to welcome a good partner into my life when the time is right*.

Instead of pressing on or giving up, let go and allow things to unfold for you. If you can, this is the greatest sign of being ready for—and welcoming—new lessons and experiences in your life. When you try to force something, you'll get trapped in a feedback loop. Surrender is the word you want to explore when it comes to life. You need to meet enough people in your life to be able to find a suitable partner. You need to know what is out there before you can know what feels right. On an energetic level, if you only set your mind on one outcome without considering alternatives, you might energetically push the right partner away. It all needs to align. Trying to force it to fall into place exactly the way you want will never turn out as you expected.

An Honest Self-Evaluation for What Comes Next

Now that you've examined and cross-examined yourself and treated your wounds, you might be ready to get back out there. But how can you truly know? Life is a constant journey, and all that matters is that we are constantly growing and gaining more capacity for unconditional love and connection. At some point, you will experience a feeling that says, "I don't mind being independently single. I'm happy with my life the way it is." This is the biggest indication that you are ready for whatever comes your way next.

What matters is finding happiness in where you are and welcoming new lessons and new experiences. And, looking back at the past and feeling nostalgia is different from wanting to travel back and be stuck in an endless time loop in that past.

After you put in the work, when looking back at the past, it should feel like looking back and not forward. The moment you can look back at the pain with gratitude is your biggest indicator that pain no longer owns you. It's a true sign that you are stepping into your power and destiny. Sometimes looking back can feel a little sad, especially when that person you once cared about is still stuck in the same place. But don't feel guilt for leaving them behind. That would have simply held you in their path. They are an immovable object, and you are an unstoppable force. This is why you have no choice but to walk with others who share a similar path, and only for as long as your paths intersect. I have met so many people who had great potential for rapid growth and healing, and yet they chose to lower their vibrations and strayed onto a *lower-level path*. But perhaps a part of their journey.

Nevertheless, the moment we let go and focus on our own path forward, we almost always bump into the right people who come along and enrich our lives. You have to be ready to let go of all attachments and simply dedicate yourself to your journey. Their journey isn't yours, even though you shared a path for a while. One must accept this. When I let go, and realised that I can't share a path with everyone at all the varying stages of my life, it was liberating, freeing. In order to continue on my path, I had to find a different tribe, a different partner, etc. Sometimes your path can sweep you up to a place where you are much farther away from what you are leaving behind, and where you start meeting people who are ahead of you. This is called catching up to where you should be, and it is always encouraging. It sounds grandiose, but sometimes leaving people behind provides hope for finding someone who is going to grow as fast as you are.

How You Know When You're Ready

I used to be drawn to party people, massive extroverts, people who were a bit more egotistic, often overcompensating for their insecurities, and covering it up with partying and drinking. That was back when I shared that vibrational path with them. The more I dropped the ego, the more I was happy just to listen and be around people. This led to desiring the company of those who were more into healthier lifestyles and outlooks, and those who might be perceived as more of introverted insightful, deathful, and interested in sharing ideas rather than drinking and partying and hiding in shallow behaviors from the depths.

We gravitate towards what we find attractive, and what finds us attractive. Someone on a different vibrational level might often not be seen as attractive. Yet, as you climb up in your vibrations, your priorities might change, such as physical looks or style seeming less important, or societal norms and beliefs no longer holding as much weight. This has to do with the feelings attached to them. You might find yourself redefining your *type*.

We attract what we project to the world. And this is not just an idea. Quantum Physics states that we attract things and people at a similar vibrational level. And, a sign of leveling up is when you find that each person you meet seems slightly more impressive than the last. So, trust your instincts instead of trying to be logical when reengaging in romantic pursuits. Now that you are practiced at listening to the parts of yourself, the varying energy systems of your body and subconscious, and being in tune with the emotions you experience, you can openly listen and hear what the sensations of your body are telling you, and having a strong intuition for what *feels* right. And you couldn't have this superpower without gratitude for the times of your life that are marked by pain.

Sometimes we need to revisit a situation to be able to see how much we don't want to be in it. This means not losing ground and maintaining your higher vibrational level while briefly visiting a lower one. You know the feeling when you have been living in a different place or country and you go home for a holiday and everything seems the same yet is much different? Maybe it no longer feels like home because you built a better life elsewhere? Or being in that place used to feel comforting and now it's just not that fun? Or, meeting up with friends from your past, and they're all still hanging around the same bar, and still throwing the same old parties, and you no longer feel like you belong?

Personally, I prefer more serene and sober spaces and people now. Connection is the experience I am longing for. It's common to feel bored by things we've outgrown and left behind. You are no longer attached to them, and they are in the past. Your experience informs through the contrast of where you've come from and where you are going, from where you were and where you are. It's spoken through your inner voices and what they tell you when looking back versus looking forward. If you are looking back and want to go back, then backward is where you are standing. If you are looking forward, and are feeling impatient and expect to already be standing in the future, then you need to focus on where you are standing, and why that place is important right now. But, if when you look back, you don't want to be there, and you look at where you are standing and are happy with your present, and you look forward and feel hopeful for the direction you are patiently heading towards, then you are ready for the next challenges that will come your way.

Exercise 15
Counting Your Blessings

To behold the gravity of what you've accomplished, write down a list of things that you have learned through this process. What are your blessings from this era? Perhaps you could even write a memoir about it. If you can talk about it or write about it without an extreme emotional reaction, then this also can be a big indicator that you have moved on. If you find that your sense of safety and your confidence are stronger than before, this is another sign. If you can impartially reflect upon it as a blessed journey, then you've reached the finish line. Where are you now? Write that down as well. Or paint a picture depicting what your new reality looks like. Perhaps you're imagining the road, redefining your style of dating, how you are approaching your choices, your spiritual path, and your new patterns. Only you can know when you are being honest with yourself, and can truly decide whether you are ready for reengaging in the dating world. Take your time and cherish what you decided to manifest in your life. Enjoy what you bring. And, when looking back at this romantic journey, look in the mirror and you will see *the one and only* who got you there.

AFTERWORD

This book was in itself a documentation of my own path towards healing. It unfolded as a meditative practice. With each chapter came a new stage of healing. At the end of this journey, I intentionally put everything I practiced and resolved to the test with intentional triggers, to see if what I'd written could hold up. So, having long removed myself from a meaningful ex-partner, I opened that emotional door again and decided to write a final letter to him. I filled that letter with love and forgiveness... for us both. And even though I wrote different iterations of this letter many times before, this was a real goodbye. What made this final letter different was it no longer symbolised losing hope for his return, but truly realizing I no longer desired it.

I compassionately closed the door. In that letter, I expressed my love for him as a human being, expressing compassion for a person with problems similar to my own. I accepted those things that kept us apart and I expressed I'm ready to let someone new into my heart, someone healthier and more compatible to share my path. I wished him the very best, despite the pain that the relationship came with.

Choosing liberation starts when you can express forgiveness and gratitude for everything that tests and challenges you, regardless of how painful. For without them, I wouldn't have learned those lessons and gained all the knowledge that came after. To embrace the goodness that comes into your life, you have to embrace the pain that got you there. Once you can do that, you are no longer letting go, but have let go and moved on. Pleasure and goodness cannot exist without pain. Without suffering, we can't fully appreciate all that love and connection have to offer, and that appreciation—for all of those blessings and creations—should remain ever present in life. What are you grateful for? Confidence, self-love, the positive boundaries you developed, your uncompromising dedication to your growth? If you can maintain your gratitude, you start to truly be a master of your romantic journey, all while prioritising your love for yourself... above all.

Thank you for joining me on this journey.

References

Australian Government (2024) Daisy App, 1800RESPECT. Available at: https://1800respect.org.au/daisy (Accessed: 30 March 2025).

Australian Government (2025) *Crisis payment, Crisis Payment – Services Australia*. Available at: https://www.servicesaustralia.gov.au/crisis-payment (Accessed: 30 March 2025).

Brass, Larisa. "GOOD HOUSEKEEPING: How the Cleanliness (or Messiness) of Your Home Affects Your Mental, Spiritual, and Physical Health." *Vibrant Life*, vol. 35, no. 2, Mar.-Apr. 2019, pp. 22+. *Gale Academic OneFile*, link.gale.com/apps/doc/A577907412/AONE?u=anon~a473a27d&sid=googleScholar&xid=48b7d6b4. Accessed 30 Mar. 2025.

Coslett, M. (2024) *Write it down, throw it away: Easing anger with paper and pen, Neuroscience News*. Available at: https://neurosciencenews.com/anger-management-writing-25885/ (Accessed: 30 March 2025).

Uniting Communities (2024) *Escaping violence payment (EVP) program, Welcome to Uniting Communities*. Available at: https://www.unitingcommunities.org/service/counselling/domestic-and-family-violence/escaping-violence-payment (Accessed: 30 March 2025).

Wesley Mission (2025) *Escaping violence payment NSW: Supporting individuals, NSW | Supporting individuals*. Available at:

https://www.wesleymission.org.au/get-support/financial-wellbeing-support/escaping-violence-payment/ (Accessed: 30 March 2025).

Wesnet (2025) *Telstra Safe Connections Program WESNET*. Available at: https://wesnet.org.au/ourwork/telstra/ (Accessed: 27 March 2025).